Case Studies
in
PEDIATRIC
EMERGENCY
MEDICINE

Edited by

Anthony J. Haftel, M.D.
Director, Division of Emergency Medicine
Childrens Hospital of Los Angeles

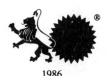

AN ASPEN PUBLICATION®
Aspen Publishers, Inc.

1986

Rockville, Maryland
Royal Tunbridge Wells

Library of Congress Cataloging in Publication Data
Main entry under title.

Case studies in pediatric emergency medicine.

  "An Aspen publication."
  Includes bibliographies and index.
  1. Pediatric emergencies—Case studies. I. Haftel, Anthony J. [DNLM:
1. Emergencies—in infancy & childhood—case studies. 2. Emergency
Medicine—in infancy & childhood—case studies. WS 200 C337]
RJ370.C37   1986   618.92'0025   86-3451
ISBN 0-87189-355-X

Editorial Services: M. Eileen Higgins

The author has made every effort to ensure the accuracy of the
information herein. However, appropriate information sources should
be consulted, especially for new or unfamiliar procedures. It is the
responsibility of every practitioner to evaluate the appropriateness
of a particular opinion in the context of actual clinical situations and
with due consideration to new developments. Authors, editors, and
the publisher cannot be held responsible for any typographical or
other errors found in this book.

Library of Congress Catalog Card Number: 86-3451
ISBN: 0-87189-355-X

Printed in the United States of America

1 2 3 4 5

Contents

CONTRIBUTORS

Nancy Schonfeld, MD
Fellow, Pediatric Emergency Medicine
Childrens Hospital of Los Angeles

Robert Morris, MD
Associate Director, Division of Emergency Medicine
Childrens Hospital of Los Angeles

Cynthia Baker, MD
Jill Kamon, MD
Chief Residents, Pediatrics
Childrens Hospital of Los Angeles

Frank Baum, MD
Misael Flores, MD
Clinical Attendings, Division of Emergency Medicine
Childrens Hospital of Los Angeles

Timothy Degner, MD
Sharon Felber, MD
Andrew Krasnoff, MD
Residents in Pediatrics
Childrens Hospital of Los Angeles

Preface

The practice of emergency medicine is demanding. Emergency department physicians are constantly being called on to evaluate sick patients and initiate therapy in an expedient, effective manner, frequently with a minimum of information. The spectrum of clinical diseases is as varied as are the patients themselves. The physician may be simultaneously handling an acute myocardial infarction in an elderly man, an ectopic pregnancy in an adolescent heroin abuser, and a febrile seizure in an infant. The successful emergency department physician is well organized, usually has mastered a systematic approach, and has learned to use all available resources (e.g., staff, laboratory, radiology, therapists) efficiently. Time is of the essence, so preplanning and anticipation are key elements of success.

The pediatric patient poses a most definite challenge to the emergency department physician. Most of these physicians do not have very much formal pediatric training and may often be intimidated by the small package that presents itself for repair. Verbal interactions if possible between the pediatric patient and the physician are generally unproductive of historical information, and thus the parent, or guardian, is the main source of the clinical history. Often the parent was not present at the onset of the disease or trauma, so this becomes second hand information, at best. Similarly, the examination of infants and small children is difficult for the practicing emergency department physician who has not mastered the "tricks" that most pediatricians use to secure confidence and cooperation in their patients.

The cases presented in this text include a wealth of basic pediatric medicine. Many common emergencies of childhood are covered, such as trauma, infectious disease, endocrine and metabolic disorders, and child abuse. The relevant available history is cited along with the initial results of the physical examination, so that the reader can develop a differential diagnosis. Cases are juxtaposed, however, to illustrate similar presentations that really manifest different disease processes.

The reader is encouraged to respond to the case presentations by thinking out, or actually writing down, a prioritized list of interventions before looking at the subsequent material.

The section entitled "Suggested Interventions" describes the method suggested by the authors for the management of each particular case. There are few absolutes in medicine, and these suggested interventions should not be construed as the only way to manage any given case but rather as the method of management that would be used in the Emergency Division of Childrens Hospital of Los Angeles.

A comprehensive review of the case is given under the heading "Case Discussion," noting pathophysiology, differential diagnosis, diagnosis, and essentials of therapy. The pharmacologic aspects of the therapy are emphasized. This case discussion serves to highlight the common pitfalls made by "adult-oriented" emergency department physicians who may not see infants and children frequently enough. These areas are stressed as often as possible.

The last section, "Suggested Readings," offers recent literature articles covering the clinical material reviewed in the case presented. Only a few articles are presented for each case discussed. This is intentional and indicates to the already busy practitioner that which is believed to be most relevant and comprehensive.

This type of format should be very useful to the career emergency department physician in approaching the management of difficult pediatric emergencies. It should likewise be useful to the pediatrician who is called on to treat emergencies in a hospital or clinic setting, in that the prioritization of interventions brings to the pediatrician the essence of current emergency practice.

Abbreviations

ABD—abdomen
ABG—arterial blood gas
BP—blood pressure
BUN—blood urea nitrogen
CBC—complete blood cell count
CNS—central nervous system
CPR—cardiopulmonary resuscitation
CSF—cerebrospinal fluid
CT—computed tomography
CVS—cardiovascular
DPT—diphtheria-pertussis-tetanus
ECG—electrocardiogram
EEG—electroencephalogram
ENT—ears, nose, and throat
EOM—extraocular muscle
ESR—erythrocyte sedimentation rate
EXT—extremities
GI—gastrointestinal
GU—genitourinary
HC—head circumference
hCG—human chorionic gonadotropin
HCO_3^-—bicarbonate
HEENT—head, eyes, ears, nose, and throat
HT—height

ICU—intensive care unit
IM—intramuscular
IV—intravenous
IVFD—intravenous, fast drip
IVp—intravenous, push
IVSD—intravenous, slow drip
KVO—keep vein open
NCAT—normocephalic and atraumatic
NEURO—neurologic
NG—nasogastric
NPO—nothing per os
OFC—occipital-frontal circumference
OPV—oral polio vaccine
P—pulse
PEEP—positive end-expiratory pressure
PERRLA—pupils equal, round, react to light and accommodation
PO—per os
RBC—red blood cell
RR—respiratory rate
S_1—first heart sound
S_2—second heart sound

SC—subcutaneous
SGOT—serum glutamic oxaloacetic transaminase
SGPT—serum glutamic pyruvic transminase

T—temperature
VDRL—Venereal Disease Research Laboratory test
WBC—white blood cell
WT—weight

Case 1

Five-day-old Male with Jaundice

CASE PRESENTATION

A 5-day-old Asian male presented to the emergency department with a chief complaint of jaundice. He was the 3.4-kg product of a full-term pregnancy, born to a gravida 2/para 1 mother by normal spontaneous vaginal delivery. The pregnancy was uncomplicated. The mother received full prenatal care from an obstetrician. Specifically, there was no history of fever, infection, or viral syndromes. The mother reports taking Bendectin®* early in the pregnancy and occasionally acetaminophen (Tylenol®), but she denies taking any other medication. The neonatal history was unremarkable, and the child was discharged home with the mother on the third day of life. The mother's puerperal course was unremarkable. She has lost the child's birth records from the hospital but recalls that "his numbers were good" and notes that he had a ruddy complexion. She can recall no laboratory tests being done.

The infant is breast-feeding 10 to 15 minutes per side every 2 to 3 hours. The mother, concerned that she "doesn't have enough milk," supplements with water every 4 to 6 hours. Over the past 24 hours she reports the child has fed less vigorously and notes only one stool today, whereas the child had been defecating after each feeding previously. Today, the grandmother saw the child for the first time and was concerned that he had jaundice. The family had not yet decided on a pediatrician, and, at the grandmother's urging, have come to the emergency department.

The child is not, by history, irritable, and has not been febrile. There has been no tachypnea, vomiting, or loose or bloody stools. The urine is light yellow, and

---

*Combined product with doxylamine succinate and pyridoxine hydrochloride.

1

the mother believes the child voids often. He is taking no medication. There is no family history of liver problems or hematologic problems, except for an uncle with leukemia. There is no family history of diabetes mellitus. The previous child, a male, has no medical problems and was never jaundiced.

A call to the hospital of birth reveals that the "computer is down" and no old laboratory results will be available for 4 or 5 hours.

Vital Signs

T: 36°C (96.8°F; axillary, variable)
P: 140 beats/min
RR: 28/min
BP: 70 mm Hg (palpable)
WT: 3.4 kg

Physical Examination

GEN: Active and alert, but obviously jaundiced neonate
HEENT: *Head:* NCAT, no cephalohematoma; anterior fontanelle, 3 × 4 cm, soft; posterior fontanelle, 1 × 2 cm, soft. *Eyes:* icteric sclera; PERRL; red reflex bilaterally. *Ears:* normal pinnae; tympanic membranes poorly seen. *Nose:* no nasal flaring or rhinorrhea. *Throat:* clear
NECK: Supple; no adenopathy; no anomalies; mongolian spot seen
CHEST: Clear without retractions
CVS: Normal without murmur
ABD: Soft; active bowel sounds; liver down 1 cm below right costal margin; spleen tip felt; kidneys not palpable
GU: Normal male
NEURO: Sucks from bottle vigorously; normal complete Moro reflex; moves all extremities symmetrically, not "jittery"
SKIN: Jaundiced without rash; extremities pink with good capillary refill

SUGGESTED INTERVENTIONS

1. Obtain blood specimens for the following studies:
   a. Bilirubin total and direct fraction, stat
   b. Hemoglobin, hematocrit,* WBC count and differential, and smear for RBC morphology

---

Note: This is to be a venous or arterial sample since capillary specimens could yield a falsely elevated hematocrit at 5 days of age.

c. Direct Coombs' test,* ABO type and Rh factor
d. One drop on a Dextrostix® (result was 80 mg/dL)
2. Obtain mother's blood for ABO type and Rh, indirect.
3. Send mother and infant to waiting room pending test results. Allow mother to breast-feed the infant if she wishes.

CASE DISCUSSION

Hyperbilirubinemia in the neonate has traditionally been a diagnosis exclusively considered by the pediatrician and family practitioner. With the increasing use of alternate birthing centers and home delivery, combined with ever earlier discharges from maternity wards, the chances of encountering such a patient in an emergency department is likely.

This patient's serum bilirubin value was 17.8 mg/dL with a direct fraction of 2.2. The blood type was O +, as was the mother's. The hematocrit was 66%. RBC morphology was unremarkable without evidence of hemolysis.

Admission for this patient is mandated on the basis of both the hyperbilirubinemia and the polycythemia. At this point an IV infusion of 10% dextrose in 0.5 normal saline at 100 mL/kg/day should be started and the parent encouraged to continue enteral feedings. Any remaining umbilical stump should be cleaned and moistened in the event umbilical catheterization should be necessary.

Admission to a facility where umbilical catheterization and exchange transfusion can be accomplished is necessitated by the increased hematocrit. If necessary, transfer to such a facility should be arranged. The decision to employ exchange or partial-exchange transfusion should be made by a neonatologist or pediatrician who is well versed in similar problems. The emergency department physician's task in this case is to determine the need for admission, or follow-up, and to order any associated tests that serve to clarify such decision making.

Hyperbilirubinemia in an infant in the first month of life is defined as a total serum bilirubin level of 2 mg/dL or greater. Values less than 2 mg/dL can be termed *physiologic jaundice* due to reduced hepatic function compared with that of an adult. The direct-reacting (or conjugated) bilirubin fraction should not exceed 30% of the total.

The danger associated with unconjugated hyperbilirubinemia in the neonate is that of kernicterus, a staining of the basal ganglia with a lipid-soluble bilirubin. This disorder is associated with hypertonicity, developmental delay, seizures, and, occasionally, death. Kernicterus was largely characterized in the 1950s by

---

*Records from hospital of birth ruling out isoimmune-mediated hemolytic disease can be substituted.

studying very ill infants with hemolytic disease of the newborn secondary to Rh factor disease. This group has declined substantially in number in recent years; considerable dispute exists in the literature as to the incidence of kernicterus. One can say with certainty that ill, premature neonates are most susceptible to kernicterus, even with bilirubin concentrations of less than 10 mg/dL. The "magic number" of 20 mg/dL has long been held as the indication for exchange transfusion for jaundice. Although incidence of kernicterus in well-appearing, term neonates (such as might present in an emergency department) is debatable, this currently remains the standard of care in most institutions.

The major causes of indirect hyperbilirubinemia can be divided into five groups: (1) increased production or extravascular location of RBCs; (2) increased rate of RBC destruction; (3) reduced conjugation or uptake of bilirubin; (4) decreased excretion of conjugated bilirubin in the bile; and (5) increased reabsorption of unconjugated bilirubin from the GI tract. A complete review of the pathophysiology of neonatal hyperbilirubinemia is not within the scope of this article, nor is it requisite knowledge for the emergency department physician who seeks to identify the infant who needs, or is likely to need, intervention. Certain laboratory tests and their significance in the workup of neonatal hyperbilirubinemia are listed below:

Total bilirubin:	Total for a given age mandates admission for observation or treatment.
Direct bilirubin:	Greater than 30% of total indicates elevation of conjugated bilirubin. Infant should be examined for any signs or symptoms of sepsis (see Case 4). Associated hepatomegaly should be indication for admission to rule out hepatic dysfunction or anomaly.
Hemoglobin/ hematocrit:	Anemia should be considered in any neonate with a hematocrit of 57% or less at 1 day of age; of 46% or less at 1 week of age; and of 31% or less at 1 month of age. Anemia should suggest acute hemolysis or breakdown of extravasated blood (e.g., cephalohematoma) in a jaundiced infant. Polycythemia is a well-recognized cause of jaundice in the neonate. Polycythemia is defined as a hematocrit of 65% or more in a 1-day old, or of 55% or more at 1 week of life. Polycythemia in the newborn should suggest dehydration or "overtransfusion" from late cord clamping or low positioning of the infant before cord clamping.

Maternal and infant blood type, Rh factor:	These identify ABO or Rh factor "set-up" children more likely to develop hemolytic disease.
Coombs' test:	A direct test on the infant identifies antibodies coating the child's RBCs; an indirect test on the mother identifies circulating antibodies in her serum.
RBC morphology:	This test is used to provide direct evidence of hemolysis. In the event of negative ABO or Rh factor workup, the physician should search for other cause (e.g., glucose-6-phosphate dehydrogenase deficiency, spherocytosis, hemoglobinopathy) by history.
Dextrostix®:	Certain etiologies of hyperbilirubinemia are associated with hypoglycemia; this is a rapid and inexpensive test, the results of which can be immediately put to therapeutic use.

Criteria for admission based on hematocrit are any value greater than 70%; any value greater than 65% with bilirubin more than 2 mg/dL, irritability, hypoglycemia, poor feeding, and "jitteriness." Criteria for admission based on the bilirubin value are shown below:

Wt (kg)	Bilirubin (mg/dL)	Age (hr)			Remarks
		24 to 48	49 to 72	>72	
	<5	Follow	Follow	Follow	Patients with values less than 5 mg/dL need follow-up, not necessarily a repeat bilirubin test.
	5–9	Follow	Follow	Follow	Patients with values more than 20 mg/dL all need admission.
<2.5	10–14	Admit	Admit*	Admit*	*These patients are
>2.5		Admit	Admit,* if evidence of hemolysis	Admit,* if evidence of hemolysis	less likely to require exchange and may be admitted to a general
<2.5	15–19	Admit	Admit	Admit	pediatric ward; all
>2.5		Admit	Admit*	Admit*	others should go to a center where exchange transfusion is feasible.

Infants with bilirubin values in intermediate ("follow") levels need to be followed at least every 24 hours to ensure the bilirubin value is not approaching a level that would require exchange. Phototherapy, therapy with light of 402 to 470 nm that converts bilirubin to a photoisomer that is cleared by the liver without conjugation, is used in an inpatient setting on patients whose bilirubin levels and age indicate they may need exchange in the near future. It is not an outpatient therapy, nor is it a substitute for exchange.

The issue of breast-feeding and its relation to jaundice is a very controversial topic. True "breast-milk jaundice" is probably related to pregnane-3α,20β-diol, which inhibits conjugation and is secreted in the breast milk. This jaundice usually arises on the 4th to the 17th day of life; it can be rather high (>20 mg/dL) and may be persistent. Since only 2% of lactating mothers produce this hormone, it is not a common cause of hyperbilirubinemia. We do not advise mothers to discontinue breast-feeding except as a provocative test for this entity. In general, infants discharged home with instructions to return for a check of serum bilirubin levels should continue to breast-feed if the mother so desires.

Any child with direct bilirubin in excess of 30% of the total bilirubin, regardless of total amount, should be admitted for the evaluation of infantile cholestasis.

SUGGESTED READINGS

Cashore WJ, Stern L: Neonatal hyperbilirubinemia. In Symposium on the Newborn. *Pediatr Clin North Am* 1982;29:1191.

Gartner LT: In Rudolph AM (ed): *Pediatrics,* ed 17, Chapter 17, "The Liver." Norwalk, Conn.: Appleton-Century-Crofts, 1981, pp 1007–1013.

Gross GP, Hathaway WE, McGaughey HR: Hyperviscosity in the neonate. *J Pediatr* 1973;82:1004.

Maisels MJ: In Avery GB (ed): *Neonatology,* ed 2., Chapter 24, "Neonatal Jaundice." Toronto, JB Lippincott, 1982, pp 473–544.

Oski F (ed): Polycythemia and hyperviscosity in the neonatal period. In *Hematologic Problems in the Newborn.* Philadelphia, WB Saunders, 1982.

Nine-day-old Male with Irritability, Jaundice, and Convulsion

---

CASE PRESENTATION

A 9-day-old white male was brought to the emergency department because he had a "febrile seizure." He was well until the previous night when he was noted to be fussy and did not have his usual good appetite. He had tactile fever and a yellow color to his nose and eyes, and he appeared less vigorous than usual. As he was being consoled, he had a short generalized seizure with his eyes deviating to the left.

A quick history revealed that the neonate was a product of a normal spontaneous vaginal delivery at 38 weeks' gestation. His mother's pregnancy was normal except for a urinary tract infection at the time of delivery. No perinatal fevers or jaundice were noted. The patient and his mother went home on the second day post delivery.

Vital Signs

T: 37°C (98.6°F, rectally)
BP: 60 mm Hg (palpable)
HR: 140 beats/min
RR: 40/min
WT: 3.3 kg

Physical Examination

GEN: Well-developed, very irritable, ill-appearing, 9-day-old male with a high-pitched cry in mother's rocking arms

HEENT: *Head:* NCAT; head circumference, 36 cm; anterior fontanelle open and tense. *Eyes:* PERRL, red reflex bilaterally; eyes do not focus on visual stimulation; sclerae mildly icteric. *Ears:* tympanic membranes clear. *Oropharynx:* dry mucous membranes

NECK: Supple; no Brudzinski or Kernig signs

CHEST: Shallow inspiratory effort when calm; moderate intercostal retractions; no rhonchi, rales, or wheezes

CVS: Normal precordium; normal S_1/S_2; regular rate and rhythm; no murmur; no gallop rhythm

ABD: Distended yet soft without increased irritability on palpation of abdomen; liver edge 2 cm below the right costal margin; no spleen tip palpated; normal noninflamed umbilicus without the umbilical cord stump

GU: Normal, uncircumcised male, with both testes in the scrotal sac

EXT: Decreased tone of all extremities; no joint swelling; no signs of inflammation; no bruises; no bony abnormalities

NEURO: Lethargic; decreased Moro reflex; no suck reflex; noninteractive with his environment; decreased knee deep tendon reflex

SKIN: Pale, mottled, cool skin with fair skin turgor; no rash; no petechiae; no ecchymosis; decreased capillary filling

SUGGESTED INTERVENTIONS

1. Administer oxygen, 3 L/min via nasal prongs.
2. Place on cardiac monitor, Doppler vital sign monitor; monitor vital signs closely.
3. Start IV with normal saline; bolus 15 to 20 mL/kg; reassess perfusion.
4. Obtain stat blood specimens for Dextrostix®, CBC, blood culture, ESR, platelet count, electrolytes, BUN, creatinine, calcium (ionized), glucose, bilirubin (total to direct ratio), blood type and hold. Dextrostix® is to rule out hypoglycemia (a cause of seizures and/or a result of sepsis). If the result of the Dextrostix® is less than or equal to 40 mg/dL, then push glucose stat as 25% dextrose in water, 0.5 to 1 g/kg (or 2 to 4 mL/kg) by IVp at the rate of 1 mL/min. *Note:* Glucose is "pushed" as 25% dextrose in water only in the neonatal period (i.e., 6 weeks and under).
5. Perform lumbar puncture. (If the patient deteriorates and is not stable, push antibiotics without lumbar puncture.) Send the tubes with CSF for the following studies:
   a. Gram stain and culture and sensitivity
   b. Glucose and protein
   c. Cell count

    d. Label and refrigerate 4th tube for other possible studies such as viral serologies, cytopathologic spin, and immunoglobulins—these are not routine tests.

6. Give ampicillin, 50 mg/kg, IV, concurrent with gentamicin, 2.5 mg/kg, IM.
7. Give phenobarbital, 10 mg/kg slow IVp for seizure control.
8. Perform suprapubic bladder tap or urethral catheterization (3 or 5 F feeding tube) of the bladder for urinalysis and culture.
9. Order chest x-ray.
10. Admit the patient.

CASE DISCUSSION

The relative incidence of purulent meningitis in the neonate has correlation to certain variables, such as perinatal complications, gestational age, and nursery experience. The relative incidence of purulent meningitis is low, but when present the morbidity and mortality rates are high. Despite improved recognition of this disease and improved initial intensive care these rates are only moderately improved. Incidence rates vary from 0.5 to 4 cases per 10,000 live births. Incidence is highest in the premature neonate and in the mother who has complications (i.e., premature rupture of membranes more than 12 hours before delivery, fever at the time of delivery, urinary tract infection, and other infections). This discussion includes infants under 3 months of age. Although meningitis is more common in the first 4 weeks of life, group B streptococcal meningitis has been seen as late as 11 weeks of life.

Organisms known to cause neonatal meningitis are (in descending order of occurrence): *Escherichia coli, Streptococcus* group B and group D, *Listeria monocytogenes, Neisseria meningitidis,* and *Hemophilus influenzae.* Hospital-acquired diseases include *Pseudomonas aeruginosa, S. aureus,* and *S. epidermidis* infections and others. It is important to recognize the distinct early-onset and late-onset diseases characteristic of both *Streptococcus* group B, and *L. monocytogenes.* In the late-onset diseases, one does not see clinical manifestations of illness in the early weeks of life. It is believed that the infant is colonized with the bacteria on surface membranes or skin.

Neonatal meningitis can be accompanied by other neonatal illnesses. Meningitis is seen in one third of the cases of neonatal septicemia. Neonatal skin infections, pneumonia, otitis media, and urinary tract infections are all associated with meningitis because of hematogenous spread (bacteremia) to the brain. Therefore, a positive culture from a site outside the CSF would be significant.

It is important to recognize that the most common signs and symptoms of meningitis in the neonate are nonspecific. Therefore, one must maintain a high index of suspicion. Findings in the history include lethargy, abnormal temperature (hypothermia or hyperthermia), poor feeding or vomiting, respiratory distress, and irritability. The classic signs of meningitis (bulging fontanelle and stiff neck) were found in only 16% in one study. Other clinical findings can include convulsions, paralysis of cranial nerves, abnormal Moro reflex, abnormal cry, and focal neurologic signs. Clinical signs of sepsis and other infections are important markers (e.g., apnea, tachypnea, tachycardia, circulatory instability, hyperbilirubinemia, distended abdomen, and swollen hot joints).

The lumbar puncture is the most specific procedure in making the diagnosis of meningitis. The CSF laboratory results can be difficult to interpret because the infant with meningitis can have normal CSF values. In one study 29% of patients with group B streptococcal meningitis and 4% of those with gram-negative bacillary meningitis had CSF white blood cell counts within the range seen in uninfected infants. Similar findings are found with the CSF protein and glucose values. The specific diagnosis ultimately depends on the demonstration of the organism on a CSF Gram stain or a positive CSF culture. In one study the CSF Gram stain was positive in 83% of infants with group B streptococcal meningitis and in 78% with gram-negative meningitis.

CSF values from neonates without CNS infections are as follows:

Test	Mean	Range
Cell count	8.4 cells/cu mm	0–32 cells/cu mm
% Polymorphonuclear leukocytes	60%	
Protein	90 mg/dL	20–170 mg/dL
Glucose	CSF glucose-to-blood ratio is 0.44 to greater than 1.00	

Blood cultures are positive in 50% to 60% of cases of neonatal meningitis. Counterimmunoelectrophoresis, limulus lysate, and latex particle agglutination may be useful in identifying the infectious agent.

Until a definitive diagnosis is made, empiric antibiotic therapy must be started in the septic, unstable infant or in the infant with cloudy-appearing CSF. In the neonate, empiric therapy consists of ampicillin and gentamicin. After admission, antibiotic therapy will be augmented to the specific pathogen and disease process identified. Penicillin G is preferred for documented group B streptococcal disease; ampicillin for enterococci, *Listeria,* or *Proteus mirabilis* infections; methicillin for *Staphylococcus* infection; and carbenicillin plus gentamicin for *Pseudomonas* infections. A combination of ampicillin and gentamicin is used against *Escherichia coli* and enterococci. One should be aware of emerging resistance of organisms (e.g., resistance of gram-negative rods to chloramphenicol and moxalactam). *H. influenzae* meningitis is presently being treated with cefuroxime alone in some centers. Other institutions are waiting to see the proven efficacy of this regimen. The hesitation is due to the emergence of resistance as seen with other cephalosporins.

Age	Possible Organisms	Antibiotic of Choice	Dosage
< 1 month	*E. coli* Group B or D *Streptococcus* *H. influenzae* *Listeria* *N. meningitidis* *S. pneumoniae*	Ampicillin plus an aminoglycoside:	50 mg/kg, IV, initial dose, then 50 mg/kg every 6 hours in infants over 7 days of age. The dosage in neonates under 7 days old is 50 mg/kg, IV, every 12 hours.
		Kanamycin	15 to 30 mg/kg/day in divided doses every 12 hours or every 8 hours
		Gentamicin	2.5 mg/kg, IM or IV, every 8 hours (neonates under 7 days old, 2.5 every 12 hours); in infants who do not respond to systemic therapy some centers recommend intraventricular administration of 1 mg every 24 hours.
		Tobramycin	Same as for gentamicin
1 to 3 months	*H. influenzae* *S. pneumoniae* *N. meningitidis* Group B *Streptococcus*	Ampicillin plus chloramphenicol	See above for ampicillin; add chloramphenicol, 25 mg/kg, IV, every 6 hours
		or cefuroxime	50 mg/kg, IV, every 6 hours

The Neonatal Meningitis Cooperative Study Group was unable to demonstrate a significant improvement in morbidity and mortality rates for infants with gram-negative bacillary meningitis treated with intrathecal gentamicin or with direct daily instillation of gentamicin into the ventricles. There are some centers that continue to advocate the use of intraventricular gentamicin despite these findings.

The CSF should be reexamined 24 to 48 hours after initiation of therapy to help assess efficacy of antibiotic treatment.

Once the pathogen has been identified and the susceptibility studies are available, the single drug or combination of drugs that is most effective should be used. Duration of therapy for neonatal meningitis is dependent on the length of time necessary to sterilize the CNS. Usually the systemic treatment for gram-positive streptococcal meningitis is about 2 weeks; for gram-negative bacillary meningitis it is 3 weeks or longer.

General supportive therapy is important in caring for these infants. Disturbance of fluid and electrolyte balance is common. In the first days of illness inappropriate antidiuretic hormone secretion can lead to fluid retention, hyponatremia, seizures, and cerebral edema. Ventilatory assistance may be necessary. Careful monitoring of vital signs is crucial, especially the blood pressure. As in sepsis, fresh whole blood or frozen plasma is transfused as a means of providing nonspecific factors of host resistance.

Fluids are generally restricted to two thirds of daily maintenance levels (see Case 18). Hypotension, however, should be treated initially with normal saline boluses (15 to 20 mL/kg) and if refractory to volume, a vasopressor such as dopamine (1 to 20 μg/kg/min) is added.

Seizures caused by significant hyponatremia (Na level $<$ 115 mEq/L) are generally treated by IV pushes of 3% saline,* calculated as follows:

$$\frac{(135 - [Na]) \times 0.6 \times WT(kg)}{4} = \text{mEq Na}^+ \text{ to be pushed}$$

where [Na] = serum sodium level.

The mortality of neonatal meningitis remains high with a range of 20% to 50% depending on the etiologic agent, predisposing risk factors, and general or intensive supportive care provided by the medical staff and available equipment. The acute complications include communicating or noncommunicating hydrocephalus, subdural effusions, ventriculitis, deafness, blindness, gross retardation, and perceptual difficulties. Forty to 50% of survivors will have some evidence of neurologic damage.

The neonate in this case study grew group B *Streptococcus* from blood and CSF. Antibiotic therapy was continued for 2 weeks. He appeared to have no sequelae at his 6-month well-baby checkup.

SUGGESTED READINGS

Dorman PH, Banker BQ: Neonatal meningitis: A clinical and pathological study of 29 cases. *Pediatrics* 1966;38:1.

Note: 3% saline has 0.5 mEq/mL.

McCracken GH: Neonatal septicemia and meningitis. *Hosp Pract* 1980;11:89.

Schaad VB, Drucko TR, Pfenninger AJ: An extended experience with cefuroxime therapy of childhood bacterial meningitis. *Pediatr Infect Dis* 1984;3:5.

Speer J: Neonatal septicemia and meningitis in Gottingen, West Germany. *Pediatr Infect Dis* 1985;4:1.

Squire E, Favara B, Todd J: Diagnosis of neonatal bacterial infection: Hematologic and pathologic findings in fatal and nonfatal cases. *Pediatrics* 1979;64:60.

Fourteen-day-old Female with Jaundice and Irritability

CASE PRESENTATION

A 14-day-old black female was brought to the emergency department by her mother with the chief complaint of increasing irritability, decreased feeding with a poor suck, and yellowing of the eyes. She has noted occasional spells when the infant appears to stop breathing. The child no longer attends to the mother's smile. Today the mother noted an elevated temperature.

The child was a full-term product of a normal, spontaneous vaginal delivery with no prepartum or postpartum complications. The child went home on the second day of life. She has been bottle feeding well until 2 days prior to presentation. There is some type of anemia in the family history.

Vital Signs

T: 39°C (102.2°F, axillary)
BP: 55 mm Hg (palpable)
HR: 145 beats/min
RR: 40/min
WT: 3.5 kg

Physical Examination

GEN: Mottled and slightly lethargic infant
HEENT: *Head:* flat anterior fontanelle. *Eyes:* conjunctiva clear; EOM intact; PERRLA; red reflex bilaterally; icteric sclerae. *Ears:* clear tympanic membranes. *Oropharynx:* dry mucous membranes

NECK: Supple with no nodes; no Kernig or Brudzinski signs
CHEST: Moderate intercostal retractions with fields clear to auscultation
CVS: Tachycardia without gallop rhythm or murmur; normal S_1/S_2; full pulses
ABD: Slightly distended but soft; normal bowel sounds; spleen tip palpable; liver 2 cm below right costal margin. *Rectum:* normal tone; negative for blood
GU: Normal female
EXT: No bony or joint abnormalities
NEURO: Slightly lethargic with decreased tone and poor suck; otherwise normal
SKIN: Pale with decreased capillary filling and acrocyanosis

SUGGESTED INTERVENTIONS

1. Place on cardiac and apnea monitor (if available).
2. Administer oxygen, 4 L/min, via mask.
3. Establish IV line and give normal saline, 15 mL/kg, as a bolus.
4. Obtain blood specimens for blood culture, Dextrostix®, glucose, ABGs, CBC, platelet count, electrolytes, calcium, creatinine, and bilirubin. Prepare smear for RBC morphology, sickle preparation and hemoglobin electrophoresis, and cross-match for packed RBCs (2 units initial type and cross-match).
5. Perform suprapubic bladder tap for urinalysis and culture. (Bladder catheterization may be done with 3 F infant feeding tube.)
6. Perform lumbar puncture when the patient is hemodynamically stable.
7. Order chest x-ray.
8. Give ampicillin, 50 mg/kg, IVFD, and gentamicin, 2.5/kg, IVSD or IM. Administration of the antibiotics should not be delayed if the patient is not stable enough for the lumbar puncture.
9. Admit the patient for IV antibiotic and fluid therapy and monitoring in an ICU.

CASE DISCUSSION

Bacterial sepsis remains a significant cause of morbidity and mortality in the neonate. The reported incidence of serious bacterial infections during the neonatal period (defined as less than 6 weeks) ranges from 1 in 500 to 1 in 1,000 births with mortality as high 10% to 30%. The major problem in managing neonatal infections is the identification of the infected neonate. This requires the awareness that a neonate may have a systemic illness and not be febrile or appear seriously ill.

Data suggest that almost any abnormal clinical sign or symptom may be associated with neonatal infections; however, certain findings are found significantly more often. Clinical findings of tachypnea, arrhythmia, decreased peripheral perfusion, pallor, abnormal blood pressure, abdominal distention, irritability, lethargy, and apnea are significantly associated with positive blood cultures. Other common clinical signs and symptoms found in infants suspected of having sepsis include hyperthermia or hypothermia, poor feeding, hyperbilirubinemia, diarrhea, vomiting, and cyanosis. Any history of complications with the birth or pregnancy, including premature onset of labor, prolonged rupture of membranes, and maternal fever, further identifies the neonates at risk for sepsis. Most authors agree that infected neonates over 1 week of age tend to present with fewer signs and symptoms associated with positive blood cultures, so there should be more concern for the possibility of infections in these infants.

With the nonspecific and diffuse nature of presentation of neonates with sepsis, multiple studies have looked at the use of laboratory parameters to identify the infected infant. A WBC count of less than 5,000/cu mm or greater than 15,000/cu mm is suggestive of sepsis, as is a band/neutrophil ratio greater than or equal to 0.1 to 0.2. The evaluation of a neonate who is febrile or suspected to be septic includes a CBC, platelet count, and blood culture and sensitivity. A suprapubic bladder tap or quick catheterization for urinalysis and culture should be performed, remembering that the pathogenesis of a urinary tract infection in this age-group usually represents hematogenous spread rather than ascending infection. A chest x-ray may be positive for an infiltrate in young infants even if auscultatory findings are minimal. Because of the nonspecific presentation of meningitis in this age-group a lumbar puncture is always recommended. The interpretation of the results of the tap differ slightly from those of adults and older children. Up to the age of 1 month a WBC count of as many as 25 to 30 cells/cu mm may be normal. Neonates also have higher CSF protein and glucose values. Additional studies such as a Gram stain and culture of pustules, ABGs if there is evidence of respiratory distress or acidosis, abdominal films for suspected necrotizing enterocolitis, and tympanocentesis if otitis media is present may be required, depending on the patient. Septic infants may also present with hypoglycemia, hypocalcemia, and disseminated intravascular coagulation.

Neonates acquire viral illnesses, but the onus is on the examiner to rule out a bacterial infection in view of the high morbidity and mortality. Group B *Streptococcus* and *Escherichia coli* together account for about 70% of cases of neonatal septicemia and meningitis. These infections are primarily acquired from the maternal intestinal and genital tracts or from the nursery. Other causes of sepsis and meningitis in the neonate include *Listeria monocytogenes,* gram-negative bacilli, other streptococci, *Staphylococcus aureus, Hemophilus influenzae,* and anaerobic organisms. The incidence of *H. influenzae* and *S. pneumoniae* infections in neonates has been rising over the past few years. This probably represents disease acquired at home. Neonatal infections with group B *Streptococcus* and *Listeria* can be divided into early- and late-onset forms. The early-onset forms usually present within the first 72 hours of life and are fulminant with respiratory distress and septic shock. The late-onset forms are more insidious, with onset up to 2 months after birth and variable presentations, including osteomyelitis, cellulitis, otitis media, meningitis, and pneumonia.

The age at which admission for the febrile but well-appearing neonate is mandatory remains controversial, but most authors recommend 6 weeks to 2 months. Once the infant is admitted, several treatment regimens are possible: (1) observation off antibiotics, (2) observation on antibiotics until cultures are negative, and (3) a full course of antibiotics. The decision as to which regimen is appropriate depends largely on the initial evaluation of the toxicity of the infant. A toxic-appearing neonate requires admission and a full course of antibiotics regardless of the culture results.

Most authors begin treatment in neonates with parenteral therapy with ampicillin and gentamicin, but the choice of antibiotics needs to be reevaluated depending on culture results and clinical course. *H. influenzae* infection in neonates is increasing, and most centers are reporting about a 20% resistance rate of *Hemophilus* to ampicillin. Because of differences in neonatal renal function, dosage schedules are different for patients over or under 7 days of age. The recommended dosages for ampicillin and gentamicin for neonates under 7 days of age are 50 mg/kg every 12 hours and 2.5 mg/kg every 12 hours, respectively. The recommended dosages for ampicillin and gentamicin for neonates over 7 days of age are 50 mg/kg every 6 hours and 2.5 mg/kg every 8 hours, respectively. Gentamicin levels and renal function need to be monitored during therapy. Besides antibiotics, full supportive care is necessary to maintain respiratory and cardiovascular function.

The patient with sickle cell disease is at greater risk for infection owing to a defect in the alternative pathway for complement activation, opsonization, functional asplenia, and phagocytic defects. These patients are particularly prone to infections with encapsulated organisms, especially pneumococcus. The clinical manifestations of sickle cell disease are unusual before 4 months of age, so that the affected neonate may be missed in states where neonatal screening is not mandatory. In young infants, the sickling of RBCs is suppressed by a fetal hemoglobin concentration greater than 20% maintaining a hemoglobin S content of less than 80%. The patient appears well but may have laboratory evidence of a hemolytic anemia with reticulocytosis by 10 to 12 weeks. In the past, many infants not previously suspected of having sickle cell disease have died suddenly, probably secondary to sepsis or sequestration. Morbidity and mortality from infection are high in patients with sickle cell disease, and probably all affected children under 5 years of age with fever should be admitted and subjected to aggressive IV therapy with antibiotics.

SUGGESTED READINGS

Barrett-Connor E: Bacterial infection and sickle cell anemia. *Medicine* 1971;50:97.

Gnehm H, Klein JO: Management of neonatal sepsis and meningitis. *Pediatr Ann* 1983;12:195.

Greene JW, Hara C, O'Connor S: Management of febrile outpatient neonates. *Clin Pediatr* 1981;20:375.

McCracken G: Neonatal septicemia and meningitis. *Hosp Pract* 1976;11:89.

Philip A, Hewitt J: Early diagnosis of neonatal sepsis. *Pediatrics* 1980;65:1036.

Powars D: Natural history of sickle cell disease—the first ten years. *Semin Hematol* 1975;12:257.

Spector SA, Ticknor BS, Grossman M: Study of the usefulness of clinical and hematologic findings in the diagnosis of neonatal bacterial infections. *Clin Pediatr* 1981;20:385.

Case 4

Twenty-one-day-old Male with Vomiting, Lethargy, and Abdominal Distention

---

CASE PRESENTATION

A 21-day-old male was brought to the emergency department with a 1-day history of continuous vomiting with all feedings, even with water. The mother also noted some abdominal distention and became alarmed when the child was unusually lethargic. The child was obstipated for the previous 1½ days. No history of bloody stool or emesis was elicited. The emesis was described as nonprojectile and appeared to be curdled formula; no "coffee grounds" or bile was seen. The child was on Similac® with Iron formula. Despite vomiting the child was noted to be gaining weight. The emesis was characterized as small in amount and occurring 2 to 10 minutes after every feeding. Prior to the obstipation, the stool was described as completely normal, without blood or mucus and not excessively watery.

The perinatal course was totally benign. There was no history of meconium, perinatal fever, jaundice, or respiratory distress. The child went home on the second day after delivery.

Vital Signs

T: 35.8°C (oral) (96.3°F)
P: 185 beats/min
RR: 52/min
BP: 52 mm Hg
WT: 3.65 kg

Physical Examination

GEN: Thin, well-developed Mexican-American male who seemed irritable and slightly lethargic

HEENT: *Head:* NCAT. *Eyes:* PERRLA; EOM intact; red reflex bilaterally; normal sclerae and conjunctivae. *Oropharynx:* normal; euhydrated; no enanthem

NECK: Supple; full range of motion; no nodes; negative Kernig and Brudzinski signs

CHEST: Clear, rapid rate; no retractions; no nasal flaring

CVS: Regular; no murmur, gallop rhythm, or rub

ABD: Distended; tympanitic; hyperactive bowel sounds; nontender to palpation; unable to appreciate masses due to distention

EXT: No cyanosis, clubbing, or edema

NEURO: Arousable; normal tone; symmetric Moro reflex; no pathologic reflexes; normal sensory withdrawal plantar reflex bilaterally upgoing

SKIN: Mottled; poor capillary refill; cool extremities, no cutaneous dysplasias

SUGGESTED INTERVENTIONS

1. Administer oxygen, 3 L/min via nasal prongs.
2. Place on cardiac monitor.
3. Begin Doppler continuous BP monitoring.
4. Start IV with normal saline, bolus 20 mL/kg, or 75 mL. Dextrostix® blood specimen. Reassess vital signs and perfusion.
5. Obtain blood specimens for ABGs, CBC, blood culture, ESR, electrolytes, BUN, creatinine, glucose, and type and cross-match.
6. Place NG tube; aspirate to Gastroccult®; hook to continuous suction.
7. Give ampicillin, 185 mg, IVSD, gentamicin, 10 mg IM.
8. Place bladder catheter (No. 5 F feeding tube). Obtain specimen for urinalysis, culture and sensitivity, and vanillylmandelic acid spot. Monitor urimeter output.
9. Consider lumbar puncture.
10. Order upright ''babygram'' (i.e., upright chest x-ray to include abdomen).
11. Request surgical consultation.
12. Perform abdominal ultrasonography.
13. Admit the patient.

CASE DISCUSSION

This 3-week-old infant presented to the emergency department with a combination of signs and symptoms suggesting sepsis, shock, and intestinal obstruction. The initial resuscitative events were tailored to oxygenate the patient, monitor for cardiac arrhythmia or electrolyte imbalance, initiate volume resuscitation, perform essential blood tests, look for foci of sepsis, treat the patient empirically for sepsis, and finally to rule out a surgically correctable lesion.

The bolus technique was used to assess the tentative diagnosis of hypovolemic shock, as manifested by the very poor skin perfusion and rapid heart rate. Rates up to 210 beats/min can still be considered sinus tachycardia in this young age-group. The fluid bolus was successful, and the patient showed much improved capillary refill; the mottling also improved. The pulse slowed to 140 beats/min. The IV was regulated to one and one-half times maintenance pending laboratory results.

The diagnosis of sepsis in this young age-group must always be entertained in any lethargic neonate who may or may not have a temperature. Low temperatures are classically associated with the septic infant. The finding of perfusion abnormalities further heightens the suspicion of sepsis. Other indicative signs and symptoms include seizures, staring episodes, breathing abnormalities such as apnea, jaundice, and hepatosplenomegaly.

Accordingly, this patient was "septicized" immediately following volume resuscitation. The workup for sepsis consists of a CBC, blood culture, urine culture, urinalysis, chest x-ray, lumbar puncture, and frequently a stool culture. The lumbar puncture must be deferred in this case until the child's hemodynamic status is stabilized over a period of time. We would prefer that antibiotics be pushed in a patient with suspected sepsis without a lumbar puncture, than have a child undergo lumbar puncture while unstable and suffer a cardio-respiratory arrest from that procedure. The CSF subsequently obtained after stabilization and an initial push of antibiotics will still have significant indices and will probably still grow out in culture. Latex particle agglutination and counterimmuno-electrophoresis are not affected that rapidly.

The choice of antibiotics for this 3-week-old infant follows fairly standard protocol in that the organisms of concern are enterics, GU pathogens, and group B and D streptococci, so that the most commonly prescribed combination in this age range and in this setting is ampicillin and gentamicin. There is no suggestion of staphylococcal sepsis and no prior hospitalization nor instrumentation, so that methicillin (or nafcillin) was not indicated. Dosing is straightforward in that we would treat this child with ampicillin 50 mg/kg IV loading dose (total daily dosage of 200 mg/kg, in divided doses every 6 hours), and give gentamicin, 2.5 mg/kg. The choice of route for the gentamicin becomes one of strategy. If given IV, it must wait for the ampicillin infusions, whereas if it is given IM, it can be done concurrently. Therefore, give the ampicillin IVSD at the *same* time the gentamicin is given IM. It is the age and renal function that determine subsequent dosing intervals, but all patients are given 2.5 mg/kg of gentamicin initially. As long as the patient is normotensive with good perfusion, IM injection of gentamicin is virtually comparable to IV infusion, when all temporal factors are considered. Had the patient's perfusion not improved, the gentamicin would have been given intravenously.

As in most venipunctures in the seriously ill or injured child, it is a very good idea to check initial sugar with the Dextrostix® method instead of waiting 30 to 60 minutes for laboratory determination. Sepsis and protracted vomiting are well associated with hypoglycemia. This patient's initial Dextrostix® result was 60 to 90 mg/dL.

An NG tube was placed to decompress the GI tract. The physical examination was suggestive of intestinal obstruction. The use of an NG tube is important in preventing aspiration and ameliorating against intestinal distention and perforation. Also, the character of the aspirant can assist in the identification of the disease process (e.g., bloody, bilious, feculent, "coffee grounds"). The tube should be hooked to low continuous suction and intake and output recorded appropriately.

A bladder catheter was placed to obtain urine for routine urinalysis and culture and sensitivity. Also, a urimeter was used to keep continuous output data: the findings of oliguria or anuria must be treated early to prevent the occurrence of acute tubular necrosis. A finding of output less than 1 mL/kg/hr should define oliguria. With good volume loading first, a subsequent dose of 1 mg/kg of furosemide (Lasix®) can be tried to increase urine flow rate. In small infants we favor the passage of No. 3 or No. 5 F feeding tubes, which is relatively easy and atraumatic to the urethra. The physician of record also sent the initial urine specimen off to test for vanillylmandelic acid (VMA) spot as a screen for possible abdominal neuroblastoma, which is one of the more common tumor masses presenting in this age range.

Neither the NG aspirant nor the urine was grossly bloody, nor was the "dipstick" test positive for occult blood. Similarly, the gastric aspirant was not bilious or feculent.

A portable "babygram" was obtained next. One of the nice aspects of the small child is the ability to obtain both upright abdominal and chest views on one plate. These are the most sensitive for free intraperitoneal air. The child should be hemodynamically stable before being held upright. Vital signs should be repeated while the child is upright.

The films in this case revealed multiple air fluid levels, a hazy increased density to the abdominal field, no free air under the diaphragm, and the suggestion of a large suprapubic mass. There was no air in the bowel wall nor was there air seen in the hepatic portal venous system. The bowel was not distended. No calcifications were seen in the abdomen. The picture was one of intestinal obstruction, or ileus, with no suggestion of perforation or septic bowel. The classic picture of necrotizing enterocolitis is air in the bowel wall and, in very serious cases, air in the portal system. The lungs were perfectly clear with no evidence of interstitial or alveolar infiltration or pleural effusion. Heart size was slightly small (decreased blood volume) with no evidence of intracardiac or extracardiac shunts. The heart configuration was normal and did not suggest any classic congenital defect. Nothing indicated congestive heart failure.

The surgeon who was consulted in the case was concerned with the possible suprapubic mass and radiograph suggestive of ascites. The majority of abdominal masses in this age range (neonatal period, birth to 6 weeks of age) are genitourinary. The diagnosis of bladder obstruction with resulting urinary ascites and probable ileus (secondary) was the leading possibility.

Other possibilities were intra-abdominal tumor such as neuroblastoma or Wilms' tumor or GI malformation such as duplication, atresia, malrotation, or webs. The absence of projectile vomiting and the picture of free intraperitoneal fluid made pyloric stenosis unlikely. Necrotizing enterocolitis was a definite possibility but was lower down on the list. The child was being treated for it anyway with IV fluid and antibiotic therapy, an NG tube, and a bladder catheter and with a surgeon in attendance.

The decision of the surgeon was to evaluate the mass and the entire abdominal cavity with ultrasonography. An abdominal CT scan would be a suitable alternate but carried more risk, owing to the use of IV contrast material.

The ultrasound revealed a very large bladder (the suprapubic mass detected on plain film) with thickened walls, a right hydroureter, right hydronephrosis, and extravasation of urine into the abdominal cavity (urinary ascites). The left kidney, collecting systems, and ureter were all within normal limits.

The child was admitted to the medical service with the tentative diagnosis of posterior urethral valves with lower urinary tract obstruction, right hydroureter, right hydronephrosis, and probable sepsis. GI ileus was secondary to urinary ascites.

Subsequent barium enema and upper GI tract films showed a completely patent unobstructed GI tract. The voiding urethrocystogram showed proximal urethral dilation consistent with posterior urethral valves. All cultures returned negative, and the child's hemodynamic status quickly stabilized. The child was maintained on antibiotics for 10 days, underwent suprapubic cystostomy on the seventh day, and was discharged home on cephalosporin prophylaxis of a urinary tract infection. Definitive urethral repair was planned in the future.

SUGGESTED READINGS

Davidson M: Malformations of the gastrointestinal tract. In Rudolph AM (ed): *Pediatrics,* ed 17. Norwalk, CT, Appleton-Century-Crofts, 1982.

Frantz ID, L'heureux P, Engel RR: Necrotizing enterocolitis (NEC). *J Pediatr* 1975;86:259.

Hendren WH: Posterior urethral valves in boys. *J Urol* 1971;106:298.

Jeffs RD: Symposium on congenital anomalies of the lower urinary tract. *Urol Clin North Am* 1978;5:1.

Case 5

Four-week-old Dehydrated Male with Projectile Vomiting, Lethargy, and Weight Loss

---

CASE PRESENTATION

A 4-week-old male presented to the emergency department with a 1-week history of vomiting, progressive weight loss, recent lethargy, and obvious dehydration. The child was the product of a normal pregnancy, labor, and spontaneous vaginal delivery and went home on the second day post delivery. The perinatal course was completely normal. The child started on formula of Similac® without Iron. He was growing and gaining weight normally. The vomiting started at the third week of life, was scant at first, but progressed to forceful, projectile vomitus of all feedings, immediately after feeding and of considerable volume. The child appeared otherwise unaffected and would return to the bottle avidly. There was no nocturnal vomiting, and the mother noted that he seemed to vomit only his feedings. The vomitus was described as clear initially but had developed a slightly "coffee ground" appearance over the 24 hours prior to admission to the emergency department. Most dramatic was the weight loss in the preceding 48 hours, which amounted to approximately 12 ounces. The child similarly had become lethargic and would refuse the bottle. At no time was the vomitus described as bilious.

On presentation to the emergency department the infant looked grossly dehydrated, was tachypneic, and had sunken eyes. Other significant history was negative; this was the first-born male in the family. The family history was similarly negative for any illness.

Vital Signs

T: 37.4°C (99.3°F, rectally)
P: 195 beats/min

27

BP: 55 mm Hg (palpable)
WT: 3.6 kg
OFC: 37 cm (50%)

Physical Examination

HEENT: *Head:* sunken fontanelle. *Eyes:* sunken; PERRLA; bilateral red reflex; normal sclerae and conjunctivae. *Ears:* normal tympanic membranes. *Oropharynx:* mouth dry; no acetone odor noted on breath; no enanthem

NECK: No mass; supple; no neck vein distention; no nodes, negative Kernig and Brudzinski signs

CHEST: Clear, rapid breathing; excellent tidal effort; no retractions

CVS: Tachycardic; regular rhythm; no gallop; no rub; no murmur

ABD: Left upper quadrant fullness; scaphoid lower abdominal quadrants; gross peristaltic waves seen from upper left toward the right stopping at midline; ? right subcostal mass; normal bowel sounds

GU: *Rectum:* sparse stool; heme 1+; normal tone

EXT: No cyanosis, clubbing, or edema

NEURO: Awake; arousable; symmetric Moro reflex; negative tonic labyrinthine and asymmetric tonic neck reflexes; normoreflexive, normal tone

SKIN: Reduced turgor; no rash; no jaundice; reduced subcutaneous fat; slight mottling; capillary refill of 2 seconds

SUGGESTED INTERVENTIONS

1. Administer oxygen, 3 L/min, via nasal prongs.
2. Place on cardiac and Doppler monitors.
3. Start IV with normal saline, bolus 20 mL/kg (i.e., 72 mL). Reassess perfusion. Dextrostix® first blood specimen: bolus 2 mL/kg of 25% dextrose in water for value less than 60.
4. Insert Foley catheter (or infant feeding tube: No. 3 or No. 5 F) in bladder; measure urine output with urimeter; order stat urinalysis and urine culture.
5. Insert NG tube; sample aspirant; send for Gastroccult®; hook to low suction; irrigate until clear if bloody or of "coffee ground" appearance.
6. Obtain blood specimens for CBC, BC, electrolytes, glucose, BUN, creatinine, calcium, ABGs, type and hold, blood culture, and ESR.
7. Order upright chest/abdomen "babygram" (portable).
8. Pull back NG tube after stomach is decompressed; place pacifier in infant's mouth; reexamine abdomen.

9. Request surgical consultation.
10. Perform barium swallow under fluoroscopy.
11. Admit the patient.

CASE DISCUSSION

This infant presented with profuse and protracted vomiting leading to dehydration, lethargy, and hypotension. The leading diagnosis in a 4-week-old male who vomits all of his feeding after every feeding, and shows no bile in that vomitus and then returns avidly to the breast is hypertrophic pyloric stenosis.

The differential diagnosis must include CNS disease such as meningitis, brain tumor, encephalitis, encephalopathy; sepsis with or without meningitis; GI obstructive disorders such as intestinal bands, atresia, webs, and duplications; primary urea cycle enzyme deficiencies such as ornithine transcarbamylase deficiency; and acute gastroenteritis.

The majority of these diagnoses can be excluded. In general, GI obstructive disorders appear early in life, in the first or second week, and are characteristically bilious, except for esophageal atresia, pyloric stenosis, or the rare disorder of supra-ampullary duodenal atresia or web. Gastroesophageal reflux can be associated with feedings but would also occur on recumbency. This child never vomited at night (unless he was fed at night). Although the neurologic manifestations of meningitis are nonspecific in this age range, this diagnosis along with sepsis must be considered by the prudent emergency department physician. CNS mass lesions are very rare at 4 weeks of age. Similarly Reye's syndrome is rare but not unheard of at this age. The finding of visible gastric peristalsis and a questionable mass in the right upper quadrant on initial examination are highly suggestive of high (gastric) obstruction. The subsequent reexamination with the stomach decompressed and the child calmed (pacifier) is crucial to locate the classic "olive"-sized mass in the right hypochondrium, lateral to the right rectus muscle. This finding almost unequivocally indicates pyloric stenosis.

Although medical management of this condition has enjoyed some popularity in the past, the preponderance of literature suggest operative management to be ideal.

This patient presented lethargic, borderline hypotensive, and with gastrointestinal obstruction. His initial management included administration of oxygen, monitoring, and IV volume repletion with full-strength crystalloid. The bolus technique of administering 20 mL/kg boluses of fluid was used and the patient's vital signs, skin perfusion, urine output, and mental status were constantly reassessed. Postural vital signs should always be done in borderline situations in which the volume status is confusing. A rise in pulse rate of 10% from supine position to upright should always suggest hypovolemia. Similarly, a reduction in pulse pressure, increase in respiratory rate, and frank drop in blood pressure are all positive signs.

The patient improved dramatically after a second 20 mL/kg bolus, and his level of consciousness improved. The Dextrostix® must be sent initially and if under 60, a push of 25% dextrose in water should be administered at 2 mL/kg. It usually takes too long for the laboratory to return the glucose value, and withholding sugar in a dehydrated, vomiting child could be disastrous. If the Dextrostix® value is in the normal or low range, initial IV therapy should be with 10% dextrose in normal saline. Urine output is a critical determinant of volume status, and generally less than 1 mL/kg/hr of output is unacceptable. Also, since sepsis was considered in the initial evaluation, a urinalysis as well as a urine culture must be ordered.

This patient's NG tube showed some "coffee-ground" material, and this is usually seen if the stenosis has caused enough obstruction and stasis to induce gastritis; generally, this does not cause copious bleeding and always improves with surgical correction of the obstruction. The maintenance of NG suction is mandatory to decompress the stomach and prevent preoperative aspiration.

Blood samples were sent to assess the degree and type of dehydration (see Case 18), to look for possible infectious etiologies, to determine acid–base status, and to type blood for surgery.

The physician next assured NG decompression of the previously dilated stomach, pulled the tube back into the distal esophagus, pacified the child with some oral device (e.g., nipple, pacifier), and then reexamined the abdomen. This maneuver will allow the hypertrophic pylorus to be palpated without the overshadowing large, distended stomach. Classically, the "olive"-sized mass is felt in the right hypochondrium 3 to 4 cm below the costal margin and immediately lateral to the lateral border of the right rectus muscle. This patient demonstrated this finding perfectly.

An upright "babygram" was obtained, capturing the chest and the abdomen. This revealed a clear and hyperlucent (dehydrated) lung field and a slightly small heart. The abdomen showed residual dilation of the stomach. The distal bowel pattern was nonspecific. No alveolar infiltrates were seen.

The electrolytes, BUN, Cr, glucose, and ABG studies revealed the following:

Na: 138 mEq/L
K^+: 4.0 mEq/L
Cl^-: 85 mEq/L
HCO_3^-: 40 mEq/L
Glucose: 65 mg/dL
BUN: 35 mg/dL
Creatinine: 1.1 mg/dL
pH: 7.55

Correct fluid and electrolyte repletion is essential prior to surgical correction. Poorly repleted infants have higher morbidity and mortality during and after surgery than do those whose preoperative state is well managed. The chronic vomiting involves fluid loss high in gastric chloride and potassium. Characteristically these infants first develop an acute metabolic acidosis from hypovolemia (mild), but it then is supervened by a more chronic metabolic alkalosis with hypokalemia. This patient was approximately 10% dehydrated by physical findings, as well as actual weight loss observed by the mother. He had the classic hypochloremic metabolic alkalosis as confirmed by electrolyte and blood gas analysis. His glucose level was just in the low normal range.

Initial fluid management was a 20 mL/kg IV push of normal saline. This initiated correction of the hypovolemia and hypochloremia. If hypotension persists, another push must be given. Following this, knowing also that the Dextrostix® was low, 10% dextrose in 0.50 normal saline could be used in place of the normal saline, and an infusion of approximately 30 mL/kg/hr, or 108 mL/hr, run for the first hour, while laboratory studies are pending. When the exact laboratory values are known the precise fluid orders can be written. This will be covered in detail in Case 18. Generally, nothing needs to be done about the alkalosis other than volume repletion; chloride therapy would not be indicated in this case. Also, a good guideline for surgery is to delay operation until volume is corrected and the bicarbonate level is down to at least 30 mEq/L. Potassium may be added once the serum potassium value is known and the child has been observed to urinate.

The surgeon must be called in early for his evaluation. We always prefer to have the consultation prior to any barium study.

The most direct method of diagnosing this disease is a barium swallow showing the narrow and stringlike elongated appearance of the pyloric channel. Also, the duodenal bulb forms a circumferential cuff around and superior to the projecting pyloric tumor mass, creating the "umbrella sign."

This child had good repletion of his fluid and electrolyte status, had a dramatically positive barium swallow, was maintained on IVs and NG suction for 24 hours, and was then electively operated on with a Fredet-Ramstedt pyloromyotomy. He did very well postoperatively and went home on the fifth day.

SUGGESTED READINGS

Benson CD: Infantile pyloric stenosis. In Ravitch MM, Welch KJ, et al (eds): *Pediatric Surgery*, ed 3. Chicago, Yearbook Medical Publishers, 1979.

Mellin GW, Santulli TV, Altman HS: Congenital pyloric stenosis. *J Pediatr* 1965;66:649.

Santulli TV: Congenital hypertrophic pyloric stenosis. In Rudolph AM (ed): *Pediatrics*, ed 17. Norwalk, CT, Appleton-Century-Crofts, 1977.

Four-week-old Female with Vomiting, Lethargy, and Shock

CASE PRESENTATION

A 4-week-old female had a 2-week history of vomiting. The emesis was nonprojectile, occurring four to five times per day. She has three to four loose stools per day without mucus or blood. She is only breast fed but is a poor feeder and has gained weight poorly. The mother has noted increased lethargy over the past 24 hours. There is no history of fever. The birth history and pregnancy history were unremarkable. She is on no medications. The family history is unremarkable.

Vital Signs

HR: 180 beats/min
RR: 35 beats/min
BP: 55 mm Hg (palpable)
T: 37.6°C (99.7°F)
WT: 3.8 kg

Physical Examination

GEN: Lethargic, poorly nourished infant
HEENT: *Head:* NCAT; sunken anterior fontanelle. *Eyes:* clear conjunctiva; EOM intact; PERRLA; red reflex bilaterally. *Ears:* clear tympanic membranes. *Oropharynx:* dry mucous membranes
NECK: Supple
CHEST: No retractions; clear to auscultation.

CVS: Regular rhythm without S_3, S_4, or murmur; decreased pulses
ABD: Soft; nontender; normal bowel sounds; no masses or hepatosplenomegaly
GU: *Rectum:* normal tone; stool heme-negative; palpable cervix. *Genitalia:* large clitoris with partial fusion of the labial folds, which are nonrugated and hyperpigmented
EXT: No bony or joint abnormalities
NEURO: Slightly lethargic; normal cranial nerves, motor responses, sensation, and coordination; tone and suck decreased; complete Moro reflex
SKIN: Mottled and poor peripheral perfusion with a capillary refill of 4 seconds; hyperpigmented areoli

SUGGESTED INTERVENTIONS

1. Administer oxygen, 4 L/min via nasal cannula.
2. Place on cardiac monitor and lead II rhythm strip. The rhythm strip showed peak T waves but no QRS or PR interval changes.
3. Establish an IV line and obtain blood specimens for a Dextrostix®, CBC, platelet count, blood culture and sensitivity, electrolytes, BUN, creatinine, glucose, calcium, ABGs, and red top to hold. The Dextrostix® was 80 to 120 mg/dL.
4. Give 106 mL (20 mL/kg) of normal saline as an IV bolus. Repeat the bolus if there is tachycardia, poor perfusion, or hypotension or if urine output is less than 4 mL/hr (1 mL/kg/hr). The minimum acceptable systolic blood pressure is 60 mm Hg. After the initial fluid bolus the blood pressure rose to 65 mm Hg/palpable and the perfusion improved. The IV fluid was changed to 10% dextrose in ⅔ normal saline at a rate of 53 mL/hr.
5. Give sodium bicarbonate, 4 mL (4 mEq) over 10 minutes, IVp (1 mEq/kg).
6. Begin glucocorticoid replacement with hydrocortisone, 25 mg, IV as a bolus.
7. Begin mineralocorticoid replacement with deoxycorticosterone acetate (DOCA) at a dose of 1 to 2 mg IM.
8. Insert urinary catheter to gravity drainage and send urine specimen for urinalysis and culture and sensitivity.
9. Obtain chest x-ray and upright abdominal x-ray.
10. Perform lumbar puncture when stable.
11. Give ampicillin, 190 mg, IVSD (50 mg/kg as a first dose).
12. Give gentamicin, 9.5 mg, IV or IM (2.5 mg/kg as a first dose).
13. Consult an endocrinologist and send blood sample for evaluation of 17-hydroxyprogesterone and other adrenal corticosteroids.

14. Admit to a pediatric ICU for close observation, correction of fluid and electrolyte abnormalities, diagnostic workup, and genetic counseling.

CASE DISCUSSION

This neonate was clinically dehydrated. On initial evaluation, the patient was lethargic with decreased perfusion, gross hypotension, tachycardia, a sunken fontanelle, and dry mucous membranes indicating a 15% (severe) dehydration. A minimal dehydration ($\leq$ 5%) is characterized by decreased tearing, dry mucous membranes, increased thirst, and minimal tachycardia. A moderate dehydration (10%) is characterized by a sunken fontanelle, sunken eyes, moderate tachycardia, and postural hypotension.

Regardless of the etiology of the dehydration and shock, immediate attention must be directed to restoration of intravascular volume and perfusion of vital organs. Whether the fluid loss is isotonic, hypotonic, or hypertonic, resuscitation should be initiated with normal saline. For patients with greater than or equal to 10% dehydration, normal saline at a dose of 20 mL/kg should be given as a bolus after IV access is established. If the patient remains tachycardic with decreased perfusion, is grossly hypotensive (systolic blood pressure less than 60 mmHg), or has urine output less than 1 mL/kg/hr, then another bolus of normal saline at 20 mL/kg should be given.

The electrolytes returned as follows: Na^+ = 110, K^+ = 7.4, Cl^- = 75, Bicarb = 15. Therefore, she has hyponatremic dehydration.

Hypotonic dehydration usually results from an increased solute loss in excess of water losses or from inappropriate replacement with hypotonic fluids. The differential diagnosis of hyponatremic dehydration is extensive. Most commonly it results from GI losses secondary to diarrhea and vomiting. In neonates, vomiting, diarrhea, and decreased feeding are all very nonspecific signs and symptoms and can occur with a wide variety of disorders. Sepsis in the neonate often is accompanied by GI disturbances. The possibility of sepsis in this patient cannot be ruled out, and the initiation of antibiotic therapy with ampicillin (50 mg/kg IV) and gentamicin (2.5 mg/kg IV or IM) is mandatory. Fever is a very inconsistent finding in neonates with sepsis. A CBC, platelet count, blood culture and sensitivity, urine culture, chest x-ray, and lumbar puncture when stable should be obtained to investigate the possibility of sepsis. Allergy to cow's milk may present as a history of vomiting and diarrhea and shock in the young infant. Usually there is a history of bloody stools. Milk allergy is unlikely in this breast-fed infant with heme-negative stools. Also, in the differential diagnosis is intestinal obstruction such as pyloric stenosis. The vomiting with pyloric stenosis is projectile. The child is usually very hungry. A hypochloremic hypokalemic metabolic alkalosis is the usual electrolyte abnormality, not hyperkalemia. An upright abdominal film may also help to rule out pyloric stenosis or other intestinal obstruction. Necrotizing enterocolitis may present as diarrhea, vomiting, and sepsis but is usually accompanied by thrombocytopenia, heme-positive stools, and pneumatosis intestinales. A patient with renal tubular acidosis may present with a hyponatremic dehydration. A urinalysis and comparison of the urine and serum pHs may aid in making the diagnosis. Included in the differential diagnosis of a hyponatremic dehydration is third spacing with ascites or burns, but there was no evidence of this in this patient. The most likely diagnosis based on the presence of a hyponatremic dehydration, hyperkalemia, and ambiguous genitalia would be congenital adrenal hyperplasia.

Hyperkalemia in patients with congenital adrenal hyperplasia is secondary to mineralocorticoid deficiency and sodium losses. The differential of hyperkalemia includes pseudohyperkalemia secondary to hemolysis and elevated WBC count or thrombocytosis. Commonly, the serum potassium value is elevated secondary to acidosis and the transcellular movement of potassium cations. This does not reflect a total body potassium excess; in fact, the patient may have a total body potassium deficit as seen in patients with diabetic ketoacidosis. The signs of hyperkalemia include weakness, lethargy, decreased intestinal peristalsis, and most importantly, cardiac arrhythmias. The earliest change seen in the ECG is peaked T waves followed by widening of the QRS complex and lengthening of the PR interval. These can be followed by first-degree heart block, ventricular arrhythmias, and asystole. Patients with congenital adrenal hyperplasia seem to tolerate elevated potassium levels well; however, the presence of any ECG changes requires immediate intervention.

The therapy for hyperkalemia is aimed at stabilizing myocardial membranes and forcing potassium into cells. The progression of changes in the ECG parallels the severity of the hyperkalemia. If the potassium value is less than 6.5 mEq/L and the only ECG changes are peaked T waves, restriction of potassium is probably the only therapy required. If the potassium value is greater than 7.0 mEq/L and/or the ECG has more than peaked T waves, then further therapy should be instituted. Sodium bicarbonate as a 7.5% solution (1 mEq = 1 mL) may be given at a dose of 1 mEq/kg over 10 minutes in order to facilitate the movement of potassium into the cells. Glucose (or 2 ml/kg of 25% dextrose in water in the neonate) at a dose of 1 g/kg (1 mL of 50% dextrose in water has 500 mg of glucose) followed by regular insulin at a dose of 1 unit per 5 to 6 g of glucose, IV, also facilitates movement of potassium into cells. Glucose and insulin should be used with extreme caution in patients with congenital adrenal hyperplasia because of the risk of exacerbating the tendency toward hypoglycemia secondary to glucocorticoid deficiency.

Calcium as a 10% solution of calcium chloride should be given to stabilize membranes if there are cardiac arrhythmias or if the serum potassium value is greater than 8 mEq/L. The dose is 0.2 mL/kg, and it should be administered slowly during constant cardiac monitoring for bradycardia. These patients are usually NPO so that sodium polystyrene sulfonate (Kayexalate®) may not be helpful. This neonate had only peaked T waves on her ECG, and the potassium value was 7.4 mEq/L; thus initial therapy with sodium bicarbonate only was begun.

Hypoglycemia is not common but can occur in patients with congenital adrenal hypoplasia secondary to glucocorticoid deficiency. A stressed neonate is even more likely to have hypoglycemia. If the Dextrostix® result is less than 30 to 40 mg/dL, the patient should receive a bolus of glucose of 0.5 g/kg IV as 25% dextrose and fluid should be administered with 10% dextrose and frequent monitoring of the Dextrostix®.

Hyponatremia is present secondary to mineralocorticoid deficiency. The severity of the clinical manifestations of the hyponatremia are dependent not only on the serum sodium level but more importantly on the rate of fall of the sodium level. Children with congenital adrenal hyperplasia develop the hyponatremia slowly so that they may tolerate lower sodium levels without developing the major signs of hyponatremia: lethargy, agitation, or seizures. The sodium deficit may be calculated by the formula:

$$\text{Deficit (mEq)} = (135 - \text{patient's sodium}) \times 0.6 \times \text{patient's weight (kg)}$$

For this patient the sodium deficit is:

$$(135 - 110) \times 0.6 \times 3.8 = 57 \text{ mEq}$$

If CNS symptoms are present, especially seizures, it is safe to correct about 25% of the deficit rapidly with 3% saline over 1 to 3 hours, being careful not to precipitate congestive heart failure or hypernatremia. This patient received about 20 mEq of sodium via the normal saline bolus and sodium bicarbonate so that even though the patient's lethargy may have been due to the hyponatremia, no further bolus of sodium was required during the initial resuscitation. The total sodium deficit should be corrected over 24 hours (see Case 18).

Often in patients with congenital adrenal hyperplasia presenting in crisis the shock is more severe than would be expected based on the history of diarrhea and vomiting. This is probably secondary to glucocorticoid deficiency. Fluid resuscitation alone will not be adequate, and glucocorticoid replacement is mandatory. A dose of hydrocortisone, 25 mg, IV in infants should be given during the initial resuscitation. Electrolyte losses can initially be corrected with saline, but the early administration of mineralocorticoids will be helpful. Deoxycorticosterone acetate (DOCA) at a dose of 1 to 2 mg IM should be administered to infants during the initial resuscitation.

The dehydration of patients with congenital adrenal hyperplasia is primarily extracellular. The extracellular space contains essentially no potassium, sodium at a concentration of 135 mEq/L, and chloride at a concentration of 100 mEq/L. The calculations for maintenance, replacement and deficit fluids, and electrolytes are shown below (see Case 18 for detailed explanation):

	Water	*Sodium*
Maintenance:	100 mL/kg/24 hr = 3.8 × 100 = 380 mL/24 hr	3 mEq/kg/24 hr = 3.8 × 3 = 12 mEq/24 hr
Replacement: Extracellular:	570 mL (15% dehydration, × 3.8 kg = 570 mL)	77 mEq (135 × .570 = 77 mEq)
Subtotals:	380 + 570 = 950 mL	12 + 77 = 89 mEq
Deficit sodium:		(135 − 110) × 0.6 × 3.8 = 35 mEq
Subtotals:	950 mL	89 + 35 = 124 mEq
Less amounts given in emergency department as "pushes":	− 106 mL	− 20 mEq
Totals	844 mL/24 hr	104 mEq/24 hr

Note: 104 mEq sodium/844 mL water = approximately 2/3 normal saline.

The usual recommendation for hypotonic and isotonic dehydration is to administer one half the calculated amount of fluid in the initial 8 hours and the remainder during the last 16 hours. Because of the risk of hypoglycemia, the dextrose concentration should be 10%. As indicated by the calculations the fluids to be administered after the initial resuscitation should be 10% dextrose in ⅔ normal saline at a rate of 53 mL/hr for the first 8 hours.

General measures that are essential for all hemodynamically compromised infants include administration of oxygen, frequent monitoring of vital signs, and insertion of a urinary catheter to gravity drainage. The urinary catheter is important as a means of assessing urine output and therefore adequacy of intravascular volume.

Congenital adrenal hyperplasia is a genetically transmitted disorder of adrenal steroidogenesis secondary to a deficiency of one of the enzymes required for the formation of cortisol and sometimes aldosterone. A 21-hydroxylase deficiency is the most common defect, accounting for over 90% of cases of congenital adrenal hyperplasia. About two thirds of the patients are able to synthesize aldosterone normally and have the non-salt-losing form, while one third are unable to synthesize aldosterone normally and have the salt-losing form. The non-salt-losing form can present in early childhood as ambiguous genitalia and accelerated growth or as a late-onset form with virilization, menstrual irregularities, and growth problems. Salt losers usually present in the first month of life not only with ambiguous genitalia and hyperpigmentation but also with dehydration and electrolyte disturbances. As a result of the cortisol deficiency there is a lack of negative feedback and hence an excessive production of adrenocorticotropic hormone (ACTH). The ACTH stimulates the abnormal adrenal glands, causing an overproduction of adrenal androgens and glucocorticoid precursors, such as 17-hydroxy-progesterone. Most salt losers, while able to produce some aldosterone, cannot produce enough to maintain a normal volume and electrolyte status. The signs and symptoms of congenital adrenal hyperplasia are related to cortisol deficiency, androgen excess, and salt and water losses.

The child with congenital adrenal hyperplasia may be identified at birth with the discovery of ambiguous genitalia, but these changes can be subtle and missed. The effects of salt wasting may not appear until 2 to 6 weeks of life. The signs and symptoms are very nonspecific. Often there is a history of chronic poor feeding, poor weight gain, vomiting, diarrhea, irritability, and lethargy. At other times the onset of vomiting, diarrhea, lethargy, and weight loss is very abrupt and associated with a viral illness. On the physical examination the predominant findings may be those of dehydration and shock as outlined above. In addition, the nipples and genitalia may appear hyperpigmented secondary to elevated levels of ACTH. A careful examination of the genitalia is important. Males with 21-hydroxylase deficiency may appear normal with only subtle changes in pigmentation and penile length. At birth the normal penile stretch length is 3.5 ± 0.4 cm and at 5 months the length is 3.9 ± 0.8 cm. Females with 21-hydroxylase deficiency appear virilized with clitoromegaly, fusion of the labial scrotal folds, and hyperpigmentation. The degree of ambiguity is quite variable, and genetic females have been identified as males at birth. The diagnosis is confirmed by assays of 17-hydroxyprogesterone and other adrenal steroids. Clot tubes for assays of these steroids should be drawn; however, treatment during a salt-losing crisis should never be withheld while awaiting results. Consultation with an endocrinologist should be obtained as soon as possible, and the patient admitted to the hospital for close observation, further correction of fluid and electrolyte abnormalities, diagnostic workup, and genetic counseling for the family. Admission to a pediatric ICU is optimal in view of the severe fluid and electrolyte abnormalities that may be present.

This child proved to have a 21-hydroxylase deficiency. She was discharged from the hospital after 10 days and is doing well on maintenance hydrocortisone, Florinef®, and sodium chloride.

SUGGESTED READINGS

Horner J, Hintz R, Luetsher J: The role of renin and angiotensin in salt-losing 21-hydroxylase deficient congenital adrenal hyperplasia. *J Clin Endocrinol Metab* 1979;48:776.

Kaplan S: *Clinical Pediatric and Adolescent Endocrinology*. Philadelphia, WB Saunders, 1982, pp 171–185.

New MI, Levine LS: An update of congenital adrenal hyperplasia. *Recent Prog Horm Res* 1981;37:105.

Case 7

Five-week-old Male with Irritability and Decreased Feeding

CASE PRESENTATION

A 5-week-old hispanic male presented with a 2-day history of tactile fever, irritability, and decreased feeding. The patient had two loose, greenish stools on the day of presentation without hematochezia or melena. There was no vomiting, rash, or cough noted, nor was there any history of lethargy or increased sleepiness. No change in the child's diet of cow's milk–based formula was made. History of exposure to ill persons and of significant travel was absent.

The patient was a full-term product of a normal, uncomplicated pregnancy and labor and was born by normal, spontaneous vaginal delivery. There were no postpartum complications, specifically maternal or neonatal fever, and the infant and mother were discharged on the infant's second day of of life. Birth weight was 7 pounds. The patient has never been ill. He has not yet been immunized.

Vital Signs

BP: 65 mm Hg (palpable)
HR: 145 beats/min
RR: 25/min
T: 39°C (102.2°F, rectal)
WT: 4.3 kg

Physical Examination

GEN: Alert, irritable hispanic male who quiets readily with feeding and sucks vigorously

HEENT: *Head:* anterior fontanelle: 2 × 3 cm, soft; posterior fontanelle: 1 × 1 cm, soft. *Eyes:* PERRLA; EOM intact; red reflex bilaterally. *Ears:* left tympanic membrane red and bulging without normal landmarks; right tympanic membrane pale pink, opaque, no light reflex seen. *Nose:* no discharge. *Throat:* noninjected pharynx

NECK: Supple; no Kernig or Brudzinski signs; shotty anterior cervical nodes

CHEST: Clear to auscultation; no retractions

CVS: Regular rate and rhythm; no murmur or gallop rhythm

ABD: Soft and nontender; no organomegaly

EXT: Good perfusion and pulses

NEURO: Alert; irritable; fixes on and follows examiner's finger; positive suck; Moro reflex; grasp

SKIN: Pink; slight mottling and acrocyanosis

SUGGESTED INTERVENTIONS

1. Obtain blood specimens for culture and sensitivity, CBC, electrolytes, glucose, BUN, and creatinine.
2. Order urine culture and sensitivity; suprapubic bladder aspiration or "quick" catheterization. (*Note:* child may spontaneously void with lumbar puncture.)
3. Perform lumbar puncture for CSF cell count, protein, and glucose determination; Gram stain; culture; consider latex particle agglutination (LPA) and/ or counter immunodiffusion (CIE).
4. Establish IV infusion line: 5% dextrose in 0.25 normal saline at maintenance of 430 mL/24 hr or 18 mL/hr.
5. Perform tympanocentesis for culture and Gram stain, by an emergency department physician skilled in the procedure, or arrange for pediatric or otolaryngologic consultation.
6. Give ampicillin, 50 mg/kg, IVSD and gentamicin, 2.5 mg/kg, initial dose IV or IM. Should clinical signs of sepsis be present (see Case 4) these drugs should be given in the emergency department; otherwise wait until all cultures are obtained.
7. Begin cooling measures (minimal clothing, tepid sponging). Give acetaminophen, 10 to 15 mg/kg every 4 to 6 hours as needed.
8. Obtain chest x-ray.
9. Admit patient to pediatric ward.

CASE DISCUSSION

Otitis media is the single most common pediatric diagnosis and, as such, represents the most common manifestation of infectious disease in infancy. One half of all infants experience this disease within the first year of life. The most common pathogens in infancy are pneumococcus and *Branhamella catarrhalis*, in addition to *Hemophilus influenzae*. Treatment is usually a 10-day outpatient course based solely on clinical examination. Antibiotic regimens of choice include ampicillin, amoxicillin, penicillin-sulfisoxazole, erythromycin-sulfisoxazole, trimethoprim-sulfamethoxazole, cefaclor, and most recently, amoxicillin–clavulanic acid.

Otitis media in infants under 6 weeks of age is a topic of continued controversy in pediatrics. The true incidence of the disease in this age-group has not yet been determined. Neonates presenting with fever of unknown source, radiographic evidence of pneumonia, or suspected urinary tract infection are generally subjected to a rigorous search for other sites of infection and prospective IV treatment with a penicillin and an aminoglycoside. Retrospective studies of septicemic neonates revealed a high incidence of concurrent otitis media, with enteric gram-negative organisms and *Staphylococcus aureus* as common pathogens. It is this suspected propensity toward enteric gram-negative infection that has led to the common-place inpatient treatment of otitis media in the neonate with a "septic workup" regimen.

Newer prospective studies have yielded conflicting results. Bland, in 1972, found nearly 90% *Staphylococcus* or gram-negative organisms and only 61% with ampicillin sensitivity. His study, all outpatients, contained 33% who had been premature. Shurin and associates and Tetzlaff and co-workers, in 1977, found *Staphylococcus* or enteric pathogens in only 10% to 18% of ear cultures, suggesting pathogenic flora more similar to that in older infants. In addition, in one study all of the patients were treated on an outpatient basis with no incidence of disseminated infection on clinical grounds.

This infant presented with a high fever and otitis. Fever of this degree is uncommon in uncomplicated otitis media. Consequently, the most conservative route is suggested, with a complete "septic workup" performed. There is no single correct approach to the afebrile infant with otitis, but conservatism dictates that otitis media in children 6 weeks of age and under be considered sepsis until proven otherwise. This is *especially* important for the emergency department physician who does not regularly see a large number of infants.

The safest and most conservative route, in any instance, is inpatient management, and we invariably opt for this route. In patients under 6 weeks of age, especially those who were premature, have high fevers, or have Gram stains of middle ear fluid showing gram-negative rods, inpatient therapy seems warranted. Certainly any question of toxicity in the patient mandates aggressive therapy.

SUGGESTED READINGS

Bland RD: Otitis media in the first six weeks of life: Diagnosis bacteriology, and management. *Pediatrics* 1972;49:187.

Marchant CD, Shurin PA: Therapy of otitis media. In Symposium on Anti-Infective Therapy. *Pediatr Clin North Am* 1983;30(No.2).

Shurin PA, Howie VM, Pelton, et al: Bacterial etiology of otitis media during the first six weeks of life. *J Pediatr* 1978;92:893.

Tetzlaff TR, Ashworth C, Nelson OD: Otitis media in children less than twelve weeks of age. *Pediatrics* 1977;59:827.

Case 8

Ten-week-old Male with Vomiting, Lethargy, and Bloody Diarrhea

CASE PRESENTATION

A 10-week-old white male was brought to the emergency department because the mother noted streaks of blood in the stool. The infant was a 3.5-kg product of a 22-year-old gravida 1/para 0 woman after an uneventful pregnancy and vaginal delivery. The child began breast-feeding and was discharged with the mother at 2½ days of age. The mother denied fever or other problems except that the infant vomited after some feedings. The mother also believed the child had become somewhat less active and more irritable.

The child appeared to be chronically ill and failing to thrive based on the poor weight gain and obvious emaciation and low body temperature. Additional history revealed that the infant weighed 8 lb., 1 oz. during his last medical checkup at 3 weeks of age. At 1 month of age the mother returned to work and switched the child to a cow's milk–based formula. The stools had been multiple, small, and soft during the breast-feeding, but within 2 weeks of the feeding switch they began to increase in volume. Since the mother was used to many stools she was not alarmed by the increase in volume until blood appeared in the stool. The infant was now having 10 to 15 large, watery stools a day.

The child was cared for at home by a live-in baby sitter, and there were not any known exposures to diarrheal illness. The child was not febrile at the beginning of the diarrheal episode and last urinated 2 to 3 hours before presentation in the emergency department.

Vital Signs

HR: 130 beats/min
RR: 25/min

WT: 3.1 kg
BP: 60 mm Hg (palpable)
OFC: 38 cm
T: 36.4°C (97.5°F)

Physical Examination

GEN: Thin infant with no subcutaneous fat and very little muscle tissue
HEENT: *Head:* anterior fontanelle normal. *Eyes:* prominent; PERRLA; EOM intact; red reflex bilaterally. *Ears:* normal tympanic membranes. *Nose:* clear. *Throat:* normal; euhydrated
NECK: No nodes palpable, supple
CHEST: Clear to auscultation
CVS: No murmur or gallop rhythm
ABD: Active bowel sounds; no masses or organomegaly
GU: *Rectum:* little resistance to the examining fifth finger; no tenderness on movement of the finger; 60 to 70 mL of liquid brown stool was passed; Heme 2 +; questionable small rectal fissure at 6 o'clock.
NEURO: Appeared listless while in mother's arms; on stimulation became irritable and cried; did not smile; poor head control and tone; reflexes + 1 in all extremities; upgoing toes; absent startle and stepping reflexes
SKIN: Pale; excoriated red diaper rash

SUGGESTED INTERVENTIONS

1. Obtain blood specimens for CBC, platelet count, electrolytes, BUN, creatinine, glucose, calcium, prothrombin time, and partial thromboplastin time, type and hold.
2. NG aspirate (result = heme −).
3. Test stool for pH and reducing substances in the emergency department. pH = 6.3 and reducing sugar = 2%.
4. Send stool specimen for culture, stain for polymorphonuclear leukocytes and parasites, and perform enzyme-linked immunosorbent assay (ELISA) test for rotavirus.
5. Perform urinalysis and urine culture and sensitivity.
6. Begin IV therapy with 5% dextrose in 0.25 normal saline at maintenance rate of 13 mL/hr.
7. Admit the patient.

CASE DISCUSSION

This case presents two challenges to the emergency department physician: (1) recognition that the child is chronically ill and (2) determination of the nature of the illness.

Young, inexperienced mothers may miss the importance of slow or subtle changes in their infants. By giving attention to an infant's present weight and comparing it to known previous weights the physician can assess the child's growth pattern over the previous months. Poor weight gain after the first week of life almost always means serious underlying disease.

Once the chronicity of this child's problem becomes apparent further inquiry reveals an abnormal stool pattern. The normal, small, watery stools of breast-feeding blended imperceptibly into serious diarrhea over several weeks time. The failure to thrive coincided with onset of diarrhea as evidence by the change in weight gain.

There are numerous causes for chronic diarrhea in this age-group. A partial list includes bacterial, viral, and parasitic intestinal infections; cystic fibrosis; postviral intestinal injury; and formula intolerance. Some of these are less likely because this child had no exposure opportunities (e.g., day care) and/or did not have a fever at the beginning of the illness. Cystic fibrosis often but not invariably has pulmonary symptoms, which this child did not display. The temporal relationship to introduction of cow's milk–based formula makes this the most likely diagnosis.

Infants who are sensitive to cow's milk exhibit stunted villi in their small intestine as well as colitis. Therefore, they malabsorb sugar and may also have blood in the stool. If exposure to cow's milk protein continues, the gut may become severely damaged and require months of parenteral nutrition before repair is complete. Thirty to 50% of infants who are intolerant to cow's milk are also intolerant to soy protein. Therefore, the disease is usually referred to as cow's milk/soy protein intolerance. The principal symptoms are diarrhea and failure to thrive. Although vomiting may accompany the diarrhea, it is not present alone. A mild, nonspecific elevation in neutrophils (serum) may be present. Colitis may be seen on sigmoidoscopy.

These infants require bowel rest in the hospital and then rechallenge with cow's milk formula. Some infants will respond with such severe diarrhea that hypovolemia, acidosis, and shock ensue within minutes to hours of the challenge. Therefore, these children require an IV and careful observation during the challenge. Some children respond less dramatically, but nonetheless diarrhea recurs within 24 hours. A smaller number of patients who initially tolerate the challenge will develop severe diarrhea within 7 to 10 days if cow's milk formula remains in the diet. This latter group has been designated the late responders. The latency period of this group complicated earlier attempts to define the characteristics of cow's milk/soy protein intolerance.

Once the diagnosis is established the child should remain on an elemental formula such as Pregestimil® until 1 year of age. At this time formula protein intolerance ceases to be a problem. Likewise, the diagnosis of formula protein intolerance becomes less and less tenable as a child approaches 1 year of age.

This patient was admitted to the GI service. He had a negative sweat chloride test for cystic fibrosis. His proctoscopy was positive for mild to moderate colitis; no ulcers were seen. All cultures for bacterial and viral agents were negative; Rotazyme® and stool ova and parasites were similarly negative. No proximal source of GI hemorrhage was found. The patient underwent a cow's milk allergy "challenge," which was dramatically positive, and he was discharged from the hospital on Pregestimil® formula and is now growing and gaining weight.

SUGGESTED READINGS

Bahna SL, Heiner DC: Cow's milk allergy: Pathogenesis, manifestations, diagnosis and management. *Adv Pediatrics* 1978;25:1–37.

Halpin TC, Byrne WJ, Ament ME: Colitis, persistent diarrhea, and soy protein intolerance. *J Pediatr* 1977;91:1404.

Powell GK: Milk- and soy-induced enterocolitis of infancy. *J Pediatr* 1978;93:553.

Case 9

Three-month-old Female with "Breathholding" Spell

CASE PRESENTATION

A 3-month-old white female was brought to the emergency department by her mother after an episode at home during which she stopped breathing. She was apparently well until that evening when the mother left her for 2 minutes and returning to pick her up found the infant pale, limp, and not breathing. No pulse was felt so her mother began CPR (artificial respirations), and spontaneous breathing returned within a minute.

On the way to the emergency department, the infant had a further episode. She gasped for air, her eyes rolled back for 30 seconds, and she again received CPR with spontaneous breathing within seconds. She has had an upper respiratory tract infection without fever or irritability.

The infant was the product of a 42-week gestation, with cesarean section secondary to fetal distress. Her birth weight was 6 lb., 9 oz., and she went home from the hospital after 6 days. Her diet consisted of ad lib Isomil®. Immunizations included 1 DPT and 1 OPV (1 month ago), and the infant is developmentally normal. The family history is negative for sudden infant death syndrome (SIDS) and seizures. The infant is currently receiving phenylephrine hydrochloride (Neo-Synephrine®) nosedrops.

Vital Signs

T: 36.4°C (97.5°F)
P: 150 beats/min
RR: 36/min
BP: 82/42 mm Hg

WT: 5.29 kg
HT: 56 cm
HC: 39 cm

Physical Examination

GEN: Well-developed, well-nourished female; alert, awake in no apparent distress; euhydrated, well perfused; acyanotic
HEENT: *Head:* NCAT; anterior fontanelle, 2 × 2 cm, soft, flat. *Eyes:* PERRLA; red reflexes. *Ears:* normal tympanic membranes. *Nose/Pharynx:* clear
NECK: Supple, without adenopathy
CHEST: Without retractions; clear to auscultation
CVS: Regular rate and rhythm; S_1, S_2 without murmur, gallop rhythm, or rub
ABD: Soft; positive bowel sounds; nontender, nondistended; normal liver, kidneys, and spleen; no masses
GU: Normal prepubertal female
EXT: Full range of motion; no cyanosis or edema
NEURO: Awake, alert; normal tone, muscle bulk, and strength; intact cranial nerves II through XII; no sensory deficit or nystagmus; deep tendon reflexes normal; upgoing toes; no clonus
SKIN: Normal color, without lesions (e.g., café au lait, ash leaf spots)

SUGGESTED INTERVENTIONS

1. Administer oxygen 3–4 L/min, via mask.
2. Start IV with Ringer's lactate, KVO.
3. Obtain blood specimens for CBC, platelets, ESR, blood culture, glucose, electrolytes, BUN, creatinine, calcium, magnesium (low calcium screens for possible low magnesium), and ABGs. Dextrostix®.
4. Order complete septic workup: lumbar puncture,* urine and stool culture (urine to be obtained by straight catheterization with No. 3 or No. 5 F infant feeding tube or suprapubic bladder aspiration and sent for routine urinalysis).
5. Obtain chest x-ray.
6. Admit patient for observation, apnea monitoring, and further workup to look for etiology.

---

*Tube No. 1 for culture and sensitivity and Gram stain; tube No. 2 for CSF glucose and protein; tube No. 3 for cell count; tube No. 4—label and refrigerate for other possible studies.

CASE DISCUSSION

This patient, a previously healthy infant by history, presented with a significant episode of apnea, requiring artificial respirations from her mother to abort the episode. Although she appeared well in the emergency department and her physical examination was normal, the potential seriousness of this history required prompt attention, an initial screening workup in the emergency department, and mandatory admission to a pediatric ward.

Apnea in infancy has received wide attention in recent years, both in the pediatric literature and the lay press, media, and parents' groups. By definition, apnea is the cessation of breathing for more than 20 seconds with or without bradycardia and/or cyanosis. There are three major types of apnea: central, obstructive, and mixed.

Infants with unexplained (no obvious cause) prolonged apnea are often considered to be at risk for the sudden infant death syndrome (SIDS). SIDS may be the final common pathway for a number of various illnesses, but among the vast SIDS literature the most prominent and recurring theories seem to involve apnea, hypoxia (chronic or recurrent), or both. Other theories, too numerous to mention completely, include cardiac conduction disorders (e.g., prolonged QT interval), viral infection, infant botulism or other toxins, and reaction to DPT immunizations. Literature in this area abounds, and active research is being conducted in many centers. Research includes both postmortem pathologic reports and studies involving those infants with a history of apnea or at risk for SIDS (e.g., siblings of SIDS victims).

The causes of apnea in infancy are varied and include abnormalities in the control of ventilation, seizures, intracranial hemorrhage, sepsis/meningitis, pneumonia, metabolic abnormalities (hypothermia, hypoglycemia, hypocalcemia, hyponatremia, acidosis), cardiac disease, gastroesophageal reflux, tracheoesophageal fistula, airway obstruction, anemia, hypovolemia, and drug/toxin ingestion. Due to the nature of the presentation, it may be difficult to obtain an accurate history. Witnesses (parents, caretakers) are understandably excited, upset, and often unable to remember details or temporal relationships and events. It can be difficult to distinguish/differentiate apnea from seizure activity or gastroesophageal reflux.

Since the history is often nondiagnostic for the cause of apnea, the physical examination and diagnostic workup become particularly important. Physical findings may relate to the above list of causes, however, the examination may be totally normal as in the case presented here. One must then proceed to an initial workup in the emergency department to screen for treatable causes of apnea.

A reasonable screening workup includes a full CBC, electrolytes, glucose, ABG, urinalysis, and chest x-ray. If sepsis is suspected, cultures of blood, CSF, and urine should be obtained; and if meningitis or a seizure is a likely possibility, one must evaluate the CSF. Further workup depends, in part, on the results of the above studies and is usually less urgent (i.e., can be done after admission). Most authors agree on the need for an ECG, EEG, and barium swallow. If intracranial hemorrhage is being considered, cranial ultrasound and/or a CT scan of the head may be diagnostic. Finally, sophisticated tests developed by pulmonary physiologists may be useful. These include a pneumogram (an impedance recording of respirations and heart rate) and, if required, polysomnography, which can provide information regarding the type of apnea, changes in gas exchange during apnea, sleep hypoxia/hypoventilation, and other data.

In summary, although there are abundant data, cause is found in fewer than half the cases. It is of great importance, however, for emergency department physicians to recognize the significance of true apnea in infants, to obtain careful histories, and to perform physical and laboratory examinations with thought to the possible causes. If a cause is found on initial screen (e.g., hypoglycemia, pneumonia, meningitis), it should be treated appropriately and then the patient admitted.

If no cause is found, the infant should be admitted for further inpatient workup. Pediatric consultants will then be able to effect management of the patient and try to determine whether the infant is at risk for further episodes of apnea. In those cases, CPR is taught to the parents and the infants are discharged on home cardiorespiratory monitors, with close outpatient follow-up.

SUGGESTED READINGS

Camfield P: Infant apnea syndrome. *Clin Pediatr* 1982;21:684.

Kattwinkel J: Apnea in the neonatal period. *Pediatr Rev* 1980;2:115.

Kelly D: SIDS and near SIDS. In *Pediatric Emergency Casebook,* vol 1, no. 5. Burroughs Wellcome Co, 1983.

Kelly D, Shannon D: SIDS and near SIDS: A review of the literature, 1964–1982. *Pediatr Clin North Am* 1982;29:1241–1281.

Naeye R: Neonatal apnea: Underlying disorders. *Pediatrics* 1979;63:8–12.

Valdes D: Sudden infant death syndrome: A review of the medical literature, 1974–1979. *Pediatrics* 1980;66:597.

Six-month-old Male with Wheezing and Fever

CASE PRESENTATION

A 6-month-old male presented to the emergency department "wheezing" for the first time in his life. The child has had slight upper respiratory tract symptoms for the past week. The mother became frightened when he started to cough and breathe rapidly on the morning of presentation. The child also refuses to take his bottle. There was no suspicion of foreign body aspiration. The child has had a slight fever but now has no overt respiratory symptoms except a cough. There is a family history of asthma, although no primary relatives are affected.

Vital Signs

BP: 75/45 mm Hg
HR: 144 beats/min
RR: 50/min
T: 37.2°C (99.0°F)
WT: 7.5 kg

Physical Examination

GEN: Alert infant who coughs every 5 to 10 seconds while sitting in his mother's lap
HEENT: *Eyes:* PERRLA; EOM intact; bilateral red reflexes. *Ears:* no fluid in middle ear; membranes move well. *Nose:* pale swollen mucosa with clear mucus. *Throat:* large red swollen tonsils
NECK: Several shotty nodes; no stridor; trachea midline

CHEST: Inspiratory and expiratory wheezing equal bilaterally; intracostal retractions and accessory muscle use apparent

CVS: No murmur; S_1, S_2 normally split

ABD: Negative

NEURO: Alert; moving all extremities

SKIN: Normal; no cyanosis; no eczema; no clubbing; pink nail beds

SUGGESTED INTERVENTIONS

1. Keep child in mother's lap to minimize distress.
2. Administer oxygen, 4–6 L/min, via mask or nasal cannula, which may be held at side of face if not well tolerated.
3. Administer epinephrine, 0.075 mL (1:1000), SC.
4. Reevaluate child at 10 and 20 minutes after administration of epinephrine, noting respiratory rate, wheezing, intracostal retractions, accessory muscle use, and heart rate. Ongoing therapy is based on response to this initial bronchodilator.
5. Repeat epinephrine or inhaled short-acting bronchodilator (e.g., metaproterenol, 0.01 mL/kg, nebulized in 2 mL normal saline, maximum of 0.3 mL) unless heart rate is over 200 beats/min.
6. Reevaluate child at 10 and 20 minutes.
7. Repeat bronchodilators unless heart rate is over 200 beats/min.
8. Place IV with 5% dextrose in 0.25 normal saline at maintenance rate: 100 mL/kg/24 hr = 750 mL/24 hr = 31 mL/hr. Failure to respond to three bronchodilation interventions is a definition of status asthmaticus. This child did not respond (i.e., his respiratory rate did not slow down, and his tidal airflow did not improve). Persistence of wheezing, though, is not strictly a contraindication to discharge.

    The following is a management of status asthmaticus.
9. Administer bolus of aminophylline, 35 mg (5 mg/kg), over 15 minutes if no xanthine drugs were given as outpatient.
10. Administer 1 to 2 mg/kg methylprednisolone sodium succinate (Solu-Medrol®) IVp.
11. Begin maintenance infusion of theophylline. Infusion rate for a 6-month-old child is 0.6 mg/kg/hr of theophylline. Since aminophylline is 80% theophylline, the correct infusion rate of aminophylline is:

    $$\frac{0.6 \text{ mg/kg/hr}}{0.80} = 0.75 \text{ mg/kg/hr}$$

    So for a 7.5 kg child the infusion rate would be: 0.75 mg/kg/hr × 7.5 kg = 5.5 mg/hr.
12. Obtain blood specimen for ABG analysis.
13. Obtain portable chest x-ray.

14. Admit the patient. The safest route is to admit to the ICU all patients with status asthmaticus with moderate to severe respiratory distress. If there is any question about monitoring the child's IV infusion and status on the ward, the child *must* be admitted to a pediatric ICU.

CASE DISCUSSION

A useful operating definition of bronchiolitis is wheezing in a child under 1 year of age. Not all infant bronchiolitics will continue to wheeze after 1 year of age, but many do. Likewise, few bronchiolitics respond to bronchodilators, but some do and it is advisable to consider one of these drugs.

Initially the approach is similar to the treatment of asthma. A brief history is taken and a physical examination performed with emphasis on the respiratory tract. Administration of oxygen should be begun immediately in all wheezing infants, partially to relieve their distress and partially to avoid the occasional episodes of transient cyanosis that follow administration of epinephrine to small infants.

Epinephrine is administered in the usual pediatric dose of 0.01 mL/kg of 1:1000 solution, and the response to this drug is evaluated. The maximum dose of 0.35 mL should not be exceeded. Because much of the bronchial obstruction in infants is believed to be caused by secretions rather than active smooth muscle constriction, bronchodilators usually do not have a dramatic effect. However, they often provide some relief. A child may receive as many as three doses of a short-acting adrenergic bronchodilator (e.g., epinephrine) spaced 20 minutes apart. Once an adequate response is achieved the child should be given a long-acting adrenergic bronchodilator (Sus-Phrine®, 0.005 mL/kg, maximum, 0.2 mL, or metaproterenol by nebulization) 20 minutes after administration of the last short-acting drug. An adequate response for infants is not defined as total disappearance of wheezing but rather relief of respiratory distress with evidence of adequate tidal volume and normalization of respiratory rate. An oral bronchodilator should be prescribed for the child to take as an outpatient. Since infants under 1 year of age metabolize xanthines slowly and toxic blood levels may quickly ensue, it is preferable to begin a β_2-adrenergic-agonist drug. If the child is already taking a β_2-agonist at home, a xanthine may be added using the following formula (for infants 1 year and under):

$$(0.3 \times \text{age in weeks}) + 8 = \text{mg/kg/24 hr}$$

This will determine the maximum safe daily dose. For example, a 40-week-old infant should receive a maximum dose of 20 mg/kg/day. In general, use of theophylline is not favored for children under 6 months of age.

Those infants who do not respond to bronchodilators administered in the emergency department require admission. The protocol described in the intervention section should be followed to get the patient ready for admission. A more detailed discussion of the treatment of status asthmaticus is covered in Case 30.

SUGGESTED READINGS

Ellis EF: Asthma in childhood. *J Allergy Clin Immunol* 1983;72:526.

Leffert F: The management of acute severe asthma. *J Pediatr* 1980;96:1.

Stempel AA, Mellon M: Management of acute severe asthma. *Pediatr Clin North Am* 1984;31:879.

Tabachnik E, Levison H: Infantile bronchial asthma. *J Allergy Clin Immunol* 1981;67:339.

Case 11

Six-month-old Male with Vomiting, Irritability, and Bruises

CASE PRESENTATION

A 6-month-old black male was brought to the emergency department by his parents because he was vomiting, irritable, and crying. They also found a lump on the side of his head. They stated that they had no idea how the lump got there or how long the lump had been present. When pressed for a possible explanation they said the infant had fallen several days previously to a carpeted floor from a rolling walker (a distance of 18 inches). The child has received no immunizations nor ongoing well-child care. They deny significant past medical history, sickle cell anemia, or prior hospitalizations for serious injury or illness, except hospitalization at 3 weeks of age because ''he was so small'' and had problems feeding. The infant was a 1.8-kg, 36-week product of an 18-year-old gravida 2/para 1 female.

Vital Signs

BP: 76/50 mm Hg
HR: 110 beats/min
RR: 18/min
T: 37.3°C (99.1°F)
WT: 6.5 kg (5th to 10th percentile)

Physical Examination

GEN: Alert child who smiled slightly in response to the examiner but appeared dirty and smelled of old urine and feces

HEENT: *Head:* OFC = 41 cm (just above 2nd percentile); mass over right parietal skull appeared tender to touch; the overlying skin appeared normal; fontanelle full but not bulging. *Eyes:* PERRLA; EOM intact—infant followed 180°; disk margins sharp, but two small retinal hemorrhages evident in the right eye and one in the left; no Raccoon's eyes. *Ears:* normal tympanic membranes; no hemotympanum; no Battle's sign. *Nose:* no deformity or CSF rhinorrhea. *Throat:* normal

NECK: Several shotty nodes; spine not tender; trachea in midline; no respiratory stridor

CHEST: Clear to percussion and auscultation; no palpable rib deformities, bruises, or crepitance

CVS: Regular rate and rhythm

ABD: Soft; nontender; normal bowel sounds; no masses or organomegaly; no bruises

GU: *Rectum:* Normal tone; soft heme − stool; *Genitalia:* normal uncircumcised male with both testicles down

EXT: Limbs normal and painless to inspection and palpation; bruises as noted under skin

NEURO: Passive; showed little interest in his surroundings; moved all extremities and had equal tone in all limbs with passive motion; deep tendon reflexes +2 in upper and lower extremities; downgoing Babinski response

SKIN: Bruises on right thigh, both upper arms, and anterior chest wall; several old 0.75 cm round scars (burns?) on back and right foot.

SUGGESTED INTERVENTIONS

1. Place IV with a large-bore catheter (18 or 20 angiocath) and normal saline using an adult drip chamber. Fluid is infused at a slow KVO rate. An infusion pump should always be used for any infusion in a neonate, infant, or child.
2. Obtain blood specimens for CBC, platelet count, prothrombin time, partial thromboplastin time, blood type and hold, and amylase drawn as the IV is placed.
3. Order lateral film of cervical spine (portable).
4. Perform urinalysis; dipstick immediately for blood.
5. Place NG tube with Gastroccult® test of aspirant.
6. Order skull series and skeletal survey to include chest, thoracolumbar spine, long bones, and pelvis.
7. Order neurosurgical consultation and CT scan.
8. Notify child abuse team (in absence of in-hospital team, notify state child protective agency). Discuss with parents the suspicions of child abuse.
9. Admit child to hospital.

CASE DISCUSSION

This child had retinal hemorrhages that indicated a significant head injury. Therefore, the immediate interventions included preparations for possible volume replacement, drug administration, and cerebral resuscitation. Children with open cranial sutures can pool enough intracranial blood to die of hypovolemic shock before manifesting signs of increased intracranial pressure. This is due to the "springing" of the sutures and expansion of the head to accommodate the extra quantity of blood. Therefore, careful monitoring of the child for signs of hypovolemia is mandatory.

Retinal hemorrhages may be caused by violent shaking of an infant. This shaking will also rupture the bridging veins from the cortex to the sagittal sinus, causing subdural hemorrhage. It is important to realize that there may be no external signs of trauma in these cases yet severe brain injury and hemorrhage can be present.

This child did not present with signs of increased intracranial pressure, but this may develop suddenly and rapidly. Therefore, preparations should be made for intubation and cerebral resuscitation. These children may also develop seizures, and diazepam (Valium®) and phenytoin (Dilantin®) should be readily available.

A cervical spine film should be obtained first, although significant neck injury is unusual in multiple trauma of children under 6 years of age.

Once the child's immediate medical priorities have been stabilized there is time to assess the other aspects of this child's injuries. A neurosurgical consultation and CT scan are necessary to assess possible brain injury. This child *must* be accompanied to the radiology department by a physician and nurse skilled and equipped to initiate endotracheal intubation and cerebral resuscitation if the child's condition suddenly deteriorates. Diagnostic studies were obtained to rule out occult thoracic, abdominal and skeletal injury—a standard evaluation in most child abuse protocols.

The child had both a history and physical examination suggesting child abuse. The mother was young and the child was premature. The separation from the mother for a prolonged time after birth is thought to interrupt normal maternal bonding. The fact that there was already another child in this young family may also have contributed stress. The parents did not have a reasonable explanation for the child's injury, and there were signs of old injury—bruises and the scars compatible with cigarette burns.

Once child abuse is suspected, a CBC is obtained to look for anemia. Clotting studies must be obtained to rule out the occasional "bruised" child with a clotting disorder. Even when abuse is certain the clotting system should be evaluated to avoid later questions if legal action is taken. Evaluation of the serum amylase level and urinalysis will help rule out other occult visceral trauma. Infants may sustain significant abdominal organ injury without surface bruises. Surgical consultation and abdominal CT scan with contrast media would be indicated if occult abdominal trauma was suspected.

A skeletal survey is obtained to look for fresh fractures as well as healed fractures. The presence of fractures in varying stages of healing highly suggests child abuse. An infant's bones heal very rapidly and remodel even in cases of marked deformity. Therefore there is usually no evidence of old fractures on physical examination.

Nonambulating children with normal bones do not sustain fractures by wedging them in crib slots. They also do not *usually* suffer skull fractures in falls equal to the height of the child unless the skull hits a pointed or very hard object.

While evaluating the chest film for rib fractures, the presence of pleural fluid should also be ruled out. Tears of the thoracic duct just as it enters the chest will lead to chylothorax on the left and are caused by a quick hyperextension of the spine.

Skull x-rays are evaluated for fractures as well as for sprung and widened sutures. Chronic increased intracranial pressure such as produced by a subdural hematoma causes the sutures to open, thus allowing partial dissipation of the pressure. In this case the child had a 6-cm linear fracture through the parietal bone. Linear fractures in children under 3 years of age should always be sought and identified so that they can be followed for diastasis and development of leptomeningeal cysts.

Admission to the hospital is mandatory for this child. In other selected instances admission may not be necessary and placement of the child in a foster home may be desirable. The child abuse team and child protective services should *always* be consulted to help the emergency department physician decide where to place the child.

Laws concerning when to notify the state child protective agency and police vary from state to state. If there is a child abuse team in the institution, they should take responsibility for making the appropriate notifications. In the absence of a team, it is usually best to make an immediate verbal report to both agencies and enlist their help in disposition. Written reports should follow such verbal notifications.

Lastly, the physician's suspicions of abuse must be discussed with the parents. This is often the most difficult portion of management. The reasonable anger the physician feels toward the abusing parents also complicates communication with the parents. It helps for the physician to remember that abusing parents often were abused children themselves. They tend to live in a chaotic environment and have very little support available to them. Therefore, if the physician communicates concern for the child and parents' welfare, the parents are more likely to cooperate with the medical care plan. The idea is to turn the focus of discussion away from the child to the parents' concerns and problems. Simple statements and questions such as the following can be used:

"You sure look tired."

"Having a new baby can sure be a handful. How are you coping?"

"Some babies are so hard to care for. They cry all the time. Does that sound
familiar to you?"

These questions will elicit useful information and give support to the parent. If the
mother also appears to be an abused wife, a sympathetic comment such as, "It
looks like things have been pretty rough for you," can help begin your discussion.
The physician must remember that the abusing parent only loses control for a few
seconds from time to time and spends the remainder being a "normal" parent who
is usually overcome by guilt. He must avoid getting caught in the "Who did it?"
type of interrogation.

After establishing some rapport with the parents, the physician explains the
extent of the injury and suggests the unlikely possibility that the reported circum-
stances could have created such injuries. The need for hospitalization for medical
reasons is discussed, as well as the requirement for a report to the authorities. If
hospitalization is not being considered, the need to involve protective services
must be discussed. The issue of temporary foster care is best deferred until
protective services decides if temporary placement is necessary.

SUGGESTED READINGS

Bittner S, Newberger EH: Pediatric understanding of child abuse and neglect. *Pediatr Rev* January
1981;2:197–207.

Leake HC, Smith DK: Preparing for and testifying in a child abuse hearing. *Clin Pediatr* 1977;16:1057.

Rieder KA: Parents: The unrecognized victims of child abuse. *Milit Med* 1978;143:758.

Stern L: Prematurity as a factor in child abuse. *Hosp Pract* 1973;8:117.

Case 12

Ten-month-old Male with Vomiting and Seizures

CASE PRESENTATION

A 10-month-old black male was brought to the emergency department because of loud crying and pain. The parents reported the child was well until 18 hours ago at which time the infant awoke from a nap crying and writhing in his crib. The mother attempted unsuccessfully to console the child for approximately 15 minutes, after which the child suddenly stopped crying and appeared sleepy. There were numerous episodes of alternating crying and lethargy over the succeeding time. The child had refused to drink his bottle from the beginning but had only vomited twice about an hour before arrival. There was no stool since onset of symptoms. The child voided just before leaving home.

The child has no previous history of serious illnesses or abdominal complaints. He had no fever at home, no contact with infectious diseases, no recent drug administration, and no localization of painful areas. The child had not recently been ill and was gaining weight. The child and his parents lived in the inner city of a large metropolitan area.

Vital Signs

T: 37.5°C (99.5°F)
HR: 125 beats/min
RR: 20/min
BP: 80/50 mm Hg

Physical Examination

GEN: Well-nourished child with a weight of 8.9 kg and an OFC of 46 cm (50th percentile). Initially the child was lying quietly, but then he began to scream, clutch his abdomen, and move about the examining table. After 10 minutes the child became quiet again. Bouncing the child while quiet did not appear to cause pain.

HEENT: *Head:* 0.5 × 1.5-cm open fontanelle not bulging. *Eyes: PERRLA;* EOM intact; normal fundi; clear conjunctivae; tears. *Ears:* tympanic membranes normal. *Nose:* clear. *Oropharynx:* mouth moist; pharynx normal

NECK: Supple with shotty nodes; no torticollis

CHEST: Clear without rales, wheezing, or rhonchi; percussion normal

CVS: Regular rate and rhythm; no murmur; normal S_1 and S_2

ABD: Mild distention; bowel sounds present but reduced while child was quiet; no organomegaly; no masses; no tenderness; no rebound

GU: Suggestion of a mass on the right and stool was heme trace

EXT: Moved all extremities, no areas of tenderness; no redness or swelling of joints or bone

NEURO: Used both upper extremities; equal strength in legs; deep tendon reflexes +2 at biceps, triceps, quadriceps, and Achilles' tendons; downgoing toes; grossly intact cranial nerves as judged by vision, extraocular muscles, pupils, facial symmetry, sucking a pacifier, and normal voice as evidenced by cry

SKIN: Good turgor; no rash

SUGGESTED INTERVENTIONS

1. Establish an IV line with normal saline to run KVO.
2. Order blood specimens for CBC, type and hold, electrolytes, BUN, creatinine, glucose, amylase, sickle prep, and Dextrostix®.
3. Check postural vital signs.
4. Order urinalysis.
5. Order abdominal series: upright chest x-ray, upright abdomen, flat plate of abdomen.
6. Request surgical consultation.
7. Order barium enema.

CASE DISCUSSION

This child presented with severe pain from an undetermined site. Certain causes of occult pain in childhood such as otitis media, sinusitis, and meningitis were ruled out by the history and physical examination. Likewise, bone fractures and joint inflammation were ruled out. Pneumonia was unlikely because of the absence of cough, fever, and tachypnea. An intracranial mass was partially ruled out by normal fundi, normal neurologic examination, and normal head circumference.

The abdomen remained suspicious because of the several symptoms and signs suggestive of intestinal pathology. Intussusception commonly affects infants at approximately 1 year of age. Pain and vomiting are most frequently seen with passage of a "currant jelly" bloody stool, eventually occurring 50% to 60% of the time. However, gross blood in the stool is a *late* finding, often appearing after 48 hours of symptoms. Apathy or sleepiness between bouts of pain is a very useful *early* sign of intussusception.

A right-sided abdominal mass was found on rectal examination. The absence of a mass does not rule out intussusception since even in large series of patients a mass was present only 50% to 60% of the time.

Another abdominal problem to be ruled out includes volvulus; although in this disease, most episodes happen to younger children. In addition, volvulus usually results in abdominal distention and vomiting early in the course. However, both diseases may cause intestinal hemorrhage or diarrheal stools.

Appendicitis is unlikely because there was no fever and no tenderness. This problem, although seen occasionally in infants, is rare until school age.

Initial management included ruling out impending hypovolemic shock, which may accompany any intestinal obstruction or hemorrhage. A venous line was placed, and normal saline readied in case hypovolemia developed. The postural vital signs were all normal. Consider a 10% increase in pulse rate and/or a 10% reduction in systolic blood pressure as a positive test.

The CBC provides information regarding possible infection as well as RBC status. A black child may be having his first sickle crisis, which was ruled out by the CBC and sickle prep. Lead poisoning also may present as acute abdominal pain, vomiting, and lethargy. The characteristic basophilic stippling of RBCs in this disorder can be seen on the blood smear.

Because the child was vomiting, blood samples to test electrolytes, glucose, BUN, and creatinine were drawn. A urinalysis helps to rule out renal pathology as well as inflammation near the ureter.

Radiographic studies included a standard abdominal series (i.e., upright chest x-ray, flat and upright abdomen x-ray) to look for evidence of obstruction, free air dilatation, and a mass. Plain films of the abdomen are unreliable in demonstrating masses in intussusception but may show suggestive absence of gas in the right lower quadrant.

This absence of gas was detected on the abdominal series in this child. Incidentally it was noted that there were no lead chips in the abdomen and no lead lines on the iliac crests (seen in lead poisoning).

A surgeon was asked to see the child to help decide if a barium enema could be safely used in an attempt to reduce the presumed intussusception. Children who arrive in shock, have signs of peritonitis, or have a WBC count in the range of 20,000/cu mm are at risk for bowel wall necrosis and perforation during attempted hydrostatic reduction. Additional risk factors for perforation include age under 6 months and symptoms for longer than 36 hours. A surgeon should examine the patient's abdomen before barium studies are undertaken.

A barium enema was performed that demonstrated an intussusception with a 2-cm mass acting as a lead point. The intussusception did not reduce, and the child required surgical reduction with excision of a Meckel's diverticulum—a classic lead point.

Most children who develop an intussusception at 1 year of age do not have an obvious leading point. The older the child becomes after this age the more likely his intussusception will involve a leading point. Lymphomas, duplication, polyps, hematomas, eosinophilic granulomas, and hypertrophied Peyer's patches have all caused intussusceptions. Hydrostatic reduction in these cases rarely succeeds.

Henoch-Schönlein purpura frequently causes abdominal pain, presumably because of bleeding into the gut wall. Unfortunately, these areas of hemorrhage may create a leading point resulting in an intussusception. A sudden increase in pain and/or vomiting or bloody stools in patients with Henoch-Schönlein purpura demands a barium enema.

Intussusception also occurs occasionally as a complication within several weeks of abdominal surgery.

Lastly, if the barium enema is negative and intussusception remains a possibility, an upper GI study should be done to rule out an ilioileal intussusception.

SUGGESTED READINGS

Abrahamson J, Eldar S: Childhood intussusception: Radiological documentation of a leading point determines the method of management. *Isr J Med Sci* 1984;20:76.

Ein SH, Ferguson JM: Intussusception: The forgotten postoperative obstruction. *Arch Dis Child* 1982;57:788.

Hymphry A, Ein SH, Mok PM: Perforation of the intussuscepted colon. *AJR* 1981;137:1135.

Martinez-Frontanill A, Haase GM, Ernster JA, et al: Surgical complications in Henoch-Schönlein purpura. *J Pediatr Surg* 1984;19:434.

Rachmel A, Rosenbach Y, Amir J, et al: Apathy as an early manifestation of intussusception. *Am J Dis Child* 1983;137:701.

Raudkivi PJ, Smith HL: Intussusception: Analysis of 98 cases. *Br J Surg* 1981;68:645.

White SJ, Blane CE: Intussusception: Additional observations on the plain radiograph. *AJR* 1982;139:511.

Case 13

Eleven-month-old Female with Diarrhea, Pallor, and Petechiae

CASE PRESENTATION

An 11-month-old white female presented with a 7-day history of diarrhea and a 1-day history of pallor. The patient was well until 7 days previously when she developed diarrhea. She had four to six stools per day, which were watery, but without blood or mucus. The mother was supplementing the child's usual diet with Pedialyte®, and she was taking fluids well until about 24 hours prior to presentation. Today the mother noted that the child's urine output was decreased and she appeared pale and more irritable. She voided only once in the past 24 hours. There has been no fever, vomiting, medications, travel, or trauma. No one else at home is ill. The past medical history, review of systems, and family history are noncontributory. The infant has no history of recurrent urinary tract infections. Her immunizations are up to date. Her weight 2 weeks ago was 10.0 kg.

Vital Signs

HR: 170 beats/min
RR: 40/min
BP: 120/60 mm Hg
T: 37.8°C (100.0°F)
WT: 12 kg
HT: 75 cm
Body surface area: 0.5 m²

Physical Examination

GEN: Alert, nontoxic, but pale infant

HEENT: *Head:* NCAT. *Eyes:* pale conjunctiva; PERRLA; EOM intact; flat discs; tears. *Ears:* clear tympanic membranes. *Nose:* clear nares. *Oropharynx:* few petechiae on the soft palate and moist mucous membranes.

NECK: Supple without adenopathy

CHEST: Tachypneic, but no retractions; lung fields clear to auscultation and percussion with no rales

CVS: Tachycardia without S_3 and S_4; regular rhythm; grade II/VI systolic ejection murmur at the left upper sternal border; full peripheral pulses

ABD: Soft; nontender; normoactive bowel sounds; no masses; liver extends 2 cm below the right costal margin; palpable spleen tip

GU: *Rectum:* normal tone, no gross blood; heme 1+ stool. *Genitalia:* normal prepubertal female

EXT: 1+ pedal edema but no bony or joint abnormalities

NEURO: Alert and irritable but will comfort easily; intact cranial nerves; 2+/2+ reflexes bilaterally symmetric with downgoing toes; grossly normal motor, sensory, and coordination examination

SUGGESTED INTERVENTIONS

1. Administer oxygen, 4 to 5 L/min via nasal cannula.
2. Place on a cardiac monitor.
3. Establish an IV and begin 5% dextrose in water to run at 150 mL/24 hr (6 mL/hr).
4. Obtain blood specimens for CBC, platelet count, prothrombin time, partial thromboplastin time, fibrin split products, fibrinogen, reticulocyte count, Coombs' test, smear for RBC morphology, electrolytes, BUN, creatinine, calcium, phosphorus, glucose, SGOT, SGPT, and ABGs and type and crossmatch for 2 units packed RBCs.
5. Perform urinalysis.
6. Order chest x-ray.
7. Order stool culture and stool polymorphonuclear leukocytes.
8. Request consultation with a pediatric nephrologist.
9. Admit patient.

CASE DISCUSSION

This child presents with a history suggestive of acute gastroenteritis and decreased urine output. However, her physical examination reveals good hydration with weight gain, tears, and moist mucous membranes. Clinically, there are no rales, gallop rhythm, or other evidence of congestive heart failure. She appears nontoxic with good perfusion and an elevated blood pressure, making hypoperfusion secondary to sepsis or acute blood loss also an unlikely cause of the decreased urine output. Exclusion of prerenal azotemia from dehydration, congestive heart failure, sepsis, or acute blood loss as the cause of the oliguria, coupled with the presence of hypertension and weight gain suggest that the child is in renal failure. The physical examination also reveals evidence of a hematologic abnormality, with pallor and tachycardia suggesting anemia, and purpura suggesting thrombocytopenia, vasculitis, or a coagulopathy. The differential diagnosis is fairly limited. Renal vein thrombosis may cause oliguria, thrombocytopenia, and a consumptive coagulopathy. Ninety percent of cases of renal vein thrombosis occur in children under 1 year of age, and 75% of these are under 1 month of age. The majority of cases, however, occur in children who are dehydrated. Other risk factors include acidosis, hypercoagulability, and the nephrotic syndrome. Enlarged kidneys are often palpable. Henoch-Schönlein purpura may present with GI symptoms, purpura, and renal failure developing in the first 4 weeks of illness. The purpura, however, is vasculitic and not associated with thrombocytopenia or a coagulopathy. The purpura tends to be distributed over the buttocks and the extensor surfaces of the lower extremities and be associated with joint swelling. Severe anemia is rare unless there has been significant gastrointestinal bleeding. The renal failure in Henoch-Schönlein purpura (rare) is secondary to glomerulitis. Renal failure secondary to poststreptococcal glomerulonephritis usually occurs in school-aged children and would be rare in an 11-month-old child. The course is usually characterized by renal disease 2 to 3 weeks after an upper respiratory tract illness. Cutaneous lesions, severe anemia, thrombocytopenia, and coagulopathy are unusual. Other types of glomerulonephritis such as rapidly progressing, membranoproliferative, and systemic lupus erythematosus are rare in this age-group and usually more insidious in onset. Oliguria secondary to urinary tract obstruction, trauma, reflux, or chronic urinary tract infection is usually not accompanied by diarrhea or purpura. The most likely diagnosis based on the presence of GI symptoms and evidence of renal failure, anemia, and thrombocytopenia would be the hemolytic uremia syndrome.

The hemolytic uremia syndrome is primarily a disease of infants and children under 3 years of age, although it has been described in all age-groups, including adults. It occurs in sporadic cases and in small epidemics. There is also a familial incidence, indicating some genetic predisposition. It is characterized by the triad of renal failure, thrombocytopenia, and hemolytic anemia.

The etiology and pathogenesis are not fully understood. There does appear to be a localized disseminated intravascular coagulation and microangiopathic process occurring in the kidneys. Histologic examination of the kidneys reveals that the subendothelial spaces of the glomerular capillaries are filled with lipids, RBC fragments, fibrin strands, and platelets. It is attractive to attribute the thrombocytopenia and hemolytic anemia to damage sustained while traversing the capillaries and subsequent removal by the reticuloendothelial system. This certainly occurs in the hemolytic uremia syndrome, but the localized disseminated intravascular coagulation and microangiopathic processes seem to amplify rather than initiate the events. Also implicated has been alterations in the RBC antioxidant state that predisposes it to fragmentation. In addition, there is evidence for increased platelet aggregation in part due to decreased prostacyclin levels. Cases of hemolytic uremia syndrome have followed pneumococcal infections. It has been suggested that neuramidase-producing bacteria such as *Streptococcus pneumoniae* unmask T antigens on RBCs, platelets, and glomeruli, making them susceptible to attack by anti-T-antibodies.

In the majority of cases a previously well child develops a prodromal illness. In the series published from Childrens Hospital of Los Angeles (CHLA) the most common antecedent illness (84%) was a mild gastroenteritis and in 15% it was an upper respiratory tract infection.

The gastroenteritis is usually mild, but melanoic stools and a picture similar to an acute abdomen or Crohn's disease may occur in 20% of cases. The prodromal illness is followed in 7 to 10 days by the abrupt onset of pallor, weakness, and oliguria. Some series report frequent neurologic symptoms such as lethargy, coma, and seizures secondary to hypertension, edema, or possible thrombotic events. This has not been the experience reported at CHLA. In the CHLA series, 75% presented with pallor, 36% with purpura, and 46% with hypertension. Dehydration (18%) may be present secondary to vomiting, diarrhea, blood loss, or decreased intake, but euhydration or overhydration is more common (72%). Tachycardia and tachypnea are common secondary to anemia and/or congestive heart failure. Further signs of congestive heart failure include rales, a gallop rhythm, vomiting, edema, and hepatomegaly. Hepatomegaly with or without congestive heart failure was present in 49% of patients. Jaundice was uncommon. Signs of hyperkalemia such as weakness, paresthesia, and hyporeflexia may be present. Less frequently signs suggestive of hypocalcemia such as tetany will be apparent.

Laboratory evaluation usually reveals evidence of a hemolytic anemia with a hemoglobin value less than 10 g/dL in 87% and less than 6 g/dL in 25%. The platelets are less than 50,000/cu mm in 51% of cases. The corrected reticulocyte count is greater than 2% in 92% of patients, and the smear for RBC morphology usually shows evidence of hemolysis. The direct and indirect Coombs' tests are usually negative. Factor levels, prothrombin time, and partial thromboplastin time are usually normal to increased, but there may be an increase in fibrin split products. Leukocytosis with a left shift is very common. The urinalysis usually reveals proteinuria and hematuria. Elevations of the BUN, creatinine, phosphorus, and potassium levels will depend on the magnitude of the renal damage. In addition, hypocalcemia, hyponatremia, and acidosis may be present. An ECG or rhythm strip is essential to evaluate possible hyperkalemia and hypocalcemia. Findings suggestive of hyperkalemia include peaked T waves, widened QRS complexes, and prolonged PR intervals. Electrocardiographic evidence of hypocalcemia includes prolonged QT intervals. There have also been reports of myocarditis associated with uremia and hemolytic uremia syndrome that may be evident on the ECG. A chest x-ray is indicated for evaluation of cardiac size and pulmonary edema. In children with very severe GI symptoms a barium study may reveal a diffuse colitis.

The management of an infant with hemolytic uremia syndrome requires very close scrutiny. Consultation with a pediatric nephrologist and admission to a pediatric ICU would be optimal. The majority of infants and children are fluid overloaded. The presence of congestive heart failure is an indication for dialysis. For patients like the one presented in this case study who have expanded extracellular volumes but are not in respiratory distress or hemodynamic compromise restriction of fluids to insensible losses will allow for a gradual improvement in fluid balance. Insensible losses can be calculated as 300 to 400 $mL/M^2/24$ hr. The patient will not be losing electrolytes in the urine, so usually dextrose in water is the solution of choice. To help prevent a catabolic state, a central venous line may be required to deliver concentrated dextrose solutions and hyperalimentation. A 1% to 2% weight loss per day is expected.

Hyponatremia with the sodium level less than 130 mEq/L is common in the anuric patient. Because of the risks of congestive heart failure and danger of hypernatremia, correction of the sodium loss must be done very slowly with hypertonic saline solutions. Patients with severe hyponatremia, congestive heart failure, and CNS symptoms may require dialysis. Acidosis may also be present and is an indication for dialysis. For mild cases, sodium bicarbonate may be given in a small amount IV or PO, again being careful to avoid exacerbation of the congestive heart failure with the sodium load.

ECG changes or a potassium level greater than or equal to 8 mEq/L is a medical emergency. Treatment is aimed at stabilizing the myocardial cell membranes by infusing calcium, forcing potassium into the cells with alkalinization, glucose, and insulin, and enhancing excretion with Kayexalate®. Calcium may be given as 10% calcium chloride intravenously at a dose of 0.2 mL/kg. The child should be on a cardiac monitor, and the infusion should be stopped if there is any evidence of bradycardia; it is then restarted at a lower rate when the heart rate has normalized. Sodium bicarbonate is available as a 7.5% solution with 1 mEq/mL and should be given at a dose of 1 to 2 mEq/kg IV. Glucose can be administered as 50% dextrose at a dose of 0.5 to 1.0 g/kg (1 to 2 mL/kg) IV, followed by regular insulin at a dose of 1 unit per 5 g glucose (1 unit/10 mL of 50% dextrose in water). Serum glucose levels or Chemstrips® should be followed carefully. Hyperkalemia is an indication for dialysis. Kayexalate® can be given orally or as an enema at a dose of 1 g/kg.

A blood transfusion may be required if the patient is symptomatic or if the hemoglobin value drops below 7 g/dL. Packed RBCs should be used to minimize the volume given. Also the blood should be fresh to prevent exacerbation of the hyperkalemia. The blood should be given slowly at 2.5 to 5.0 mL/kg over 4 hours with frequent monitoring of the patient's blood pressure, lung bases, and neck veins. If the potassium level is elevated, Kayexalate® should be given prior to the transfusion. The potassium level will need to be monitored with the transfusion.

Hypertension with the hemolytic uremia syndrome is usually responsive to the commonly used antihypertensives. If the patient is asymptomatic with moderately to severely elevated blood pressure, hydralazine, 0.1 to 0.2 mg/kg IV over 15 to 30 minutes, may be given and repeated every 6 to 8 hours as needed. If there is severe hypertension and evidence of encephalopathy, diazoxide, 3 to 5 mg/kg, rapid IV infusion can be used.

The indications for dialysis include persistent anuria for 48 hours, potassium levels greater than 7 mEq/L on two occasions, hypernatremia, congestive heart failure, acidosis, severe anemia, and CNS symptoms. The use of heparin, streptokinase, aspirin, and dipyridamole is controversial, and recommendations await further investigation.

This infant had an initial hemoglobin of 8.5 g/dL, potassium value of 6.5 mEq/L, BUN of 45 mg/dL, creatinine value of 4.0 mg/dL, and platelet count of 45,000/cu mm. Her chest x-ray and ECG were normal. A urinalysis revealed proteinuria and a full field of RBCs. She was observed for 24 hours while being maintained on an anuric regimen. Her urine output began to increase on the second day of admission. She required Kayexalate® twice but did not require transfusion or dialysis. She was discharged after an 8-day hospitalization and continues to have normal renal function after 6 months.

SUGGESTED READINGS

Fong JS, deChadarevian JP, Kaplan BS, et al: Hemolytic uremic syndrome. *Pediatr Clin North Am* 1982;29:835.

Lieberman E: Hemolytic uremic syndrome. *J Pediatr* 1972;80:2.

Loirat C, Sonsino E, Varga-Morena A, et al: Hemolytic uremic syndrome: An analysis of the natural history and prognostic features. *Acta Pediatr Scand* 1984;73:505.

Twelve-month-old Male with Weakness, Shortness of Breath, and Irritability

---

CASE PRESENTATION

A 1-year-old white male child was brought to the emergency department because of problems with breathing. His parents reported that for the past 3 to 4 days the child seemed to be breathing faster and lacked energy. The child was usually quite active all around the house, but for the past 2 weeks took longer and longer naps and seemed to just lie around. At first the parents welcomed the occasional respite from the child's constant movement, but they became worried when the child refused to eat.

There were no symptoms of pain, fever, vomiting, diarrhea, rash, or cough. The child was taking no medications. The parents did believe the child had become paler over the past few months. They also noted unexplained episodes of fretfulness over the past 3 to 4 months.

The child was the full-term product of a gravida 2/para 2, 26-year-old white female after an uneventful pregnancy and delivery. The child had been well since birth, and his immunizations were up to date. He ate all junior foods and took approximately 20 ounces of iron-fortified formula per day.

Vital Signs

T: 37.4°C (99.3°F)
HR: 175 beats/min
RR: 35/min
BP: 55 mm Hg (palpable)
WT: 10 kg
OFC: 49 cm

Physical Examination

GEN: Very pale child lying quietly on the examination table. Attempts to engage the child with a smile were unsuccessful.

HEENT: *Eyes:* PERRLA; EOM intact; red reflex bilaterally; pale conjunctivae. *Ears:* normal tympanic membranes. *Nose:* clear. *Oropharynx:* mouth wet; normal tonsils without erythema

NECK: Supple, shotty nodes

CHEST: Good breath sounds bilaterally; normal to percussion and auscultation; rapid breathing without retractions or accessory muscle use

CVS: Grade II/VI systolic flow murmur at apex and heard over carotid arteries; regular rhythm; point of maximal impulse felt in fifth intercostal space 2 cm to left of midclavicular line; precordium active to palpation

ABD: Nontender; normal bowel sounds; liver palpable 2 cm below costal margin; no other organomegaly or masses

GU: *Rectum:* normal tone; dark brown stool mixed with bright red blood; wet diaper. *Genitalia:* normal circumcised male

EXT: Normal without tenderness

NEURO: Moved all extremities; intact cranial nerves II through VII as evidenced by normal eye examination and symmetric face; turned toward sounds; gag reflex present if child sucked on a bottle; tendon reflexes symmetrically + 1; downgoing toes

SKIN: Pale; good turgor, mottled, poor capillary refill

SUGGESTED INTERVENTIONS

1. Administer oxygen, 5 L/min, via nasal prongs.
2. Start IV with two large-bore angiocaths in each antecubital vein. Instill normal saline. Run wide open until blood pressure and pulse normalize; then run at maintenance 40 mL/hr.
3. Place on cardiac monitor.
4. Obtain blood specimens for CBC, reticulocyte and platelet counts, electrolytes, creatinine, BUN, prothrombin time, and partial thromboplastin time and type and cross for 4 units. Also, obtain an extra clot tube and citrated tube for possible later studies.
5. Have hematocrit spun in the emergency department (result = 11%).
6. Perform urinalysis.
7. Place NG tube to look for upper GI tract blood (aspirant was Gastroccult® −).
8. Order chest x-ray (portable).

9. Perform blood transfusion, 100 mL over 2 hours.
10. Request gastrointestinal and surgical consultations.
11. Arrange for sodium pertechnetate Tc 99m scan.
12. Admit the patient.

CASE DISCUSSION

This child arrived with signs and symptoms of chronic and acute blood loss; he was hypotensive with hematochezia. Therefore, the first priority was rapid correction of the volume deficit, delivery of adequate oxygen to peripheral tissue beds, and detection of the site of bleeding. The hypotension (systolic less than 60 mm Hg in a 1-year old) was not from congestive heart failure but rather was hypovolemic. This was confirmed by the absence of a gallop rhythm, no neck vein distention, no basilar rales in the lung fields, no displacement of the point of maximal impulse, and a nonpulsatile liver. Oxygen therapy is mandatory in this hypotensive, hemorrhaging, already anemic patient.

The hypovolemic shock was treated with large-bore IV infusion of full-strength crystalloid, maintained until blood pressure normalized at least to 60 mm Hg (systolic).

After volume expansion, transfusion was the next consideration. Volume expansion with crystalloid alone in a patient with initial low hematocrit may cause hemodilution down to unacceptable values. Packed RBC transfusions would be ideal. As always, transfusion must be weighed against the risk of hepatitis, acquired immune deficiency syndrome, and transfusion reactions. In severe chronic anemia, transfusions must be administered slowly to prevent overloading the circulation. The presence of cardiomegaly and a gallop rhythm calls for even greater care. In severe anemia without heart failure, 10 mL/kg of packed cells may be administered over 1 to 2 hours. When heart failure exists 2 to 3 ml/kg may be administered over 2 hours, and if well tolerated this volume may be repeated over another 2 hours.

An NG tube is mandatory for any GI hemorrhage, to diagnose bleeding proximal to the ligament of Treitz, to initiate saline lavage if there is gastric bleeding, as well as to decompress the GI tract to prevent possible aspiration. The tube in this patient was passed, and no blood or "coffee ground" material was found. NG suction was maintained.

When the IV was placed, blood was drawn to type and cross, to characterize the type of anemia, and screen the clotting system. Specimens were obtained to test electrolytes and creatinine and for urinalysis to check renal function. The extra tubes of blood (clot and citrated) were collected in case the preliminary studies indicated the need to do specific RBC studies or other chemistries.

The CBC revealed hematocrit, 11%; hemoglobin, 3.7 mg/dL; WBC, 10,100/ cu mm with 53 segments, 1 band, 45 lymphocytes, and 1 monocyte. The reticulocyte count (corrected) was 1%. The blood smear showed hypochronic and microcytic RBCs. The indices were mean corpuscular volume (MCV) 63 and mean corpuscular hemoglobin concentration (MCHC) 28. The remainder of the studies were normal.

This patient's studies were compatible with iron deficiency, a common cause of anemia at this age. Many children develop this problem as a result of a poor diet, which usually consists of large volumes of whole milk and little additional food. There may be small amounts of chronic GI blood loss in this disease. However, this patient had a frank hematochezia. Added to this was the history of intermittent abdominal pain for several months. Several lesions with this symptom-complex may be seen at this age. Intussusception may cause rectal bleeding, but this is usually a single event and usually, but not invariably, there is significant pain. Peptic ulcer disease can cause vague pain and chronic blood loss and is responsible for approximately 11% of GI bleeding in this age-group. Duplication and Meckel's diverticulum may both contain gastric mucosa, which can result in erosion of nearby mucosa and bleeding. Juvenile polyps can cause chronic bleeding, but usually the blood is bright red and the child is over 2 years old.

This child was admitted for ongoing management of his hematochezia anemia, and further studies of the GI tract. Meckel's diverticulum is the most common cause of massive GI hemorrhage in infants. In the case of massive hemorrhage large volumes of blood may be necessary to resuscitate the child. In addition to these life-threatening hemorrhages, Meckel's diverticuli may also cause bright red rectal bleeding alternating with dark, bloody stools. Chronic bleeding with slow development of anemia is the least common presentation.

Meckel's diverticulum can also become the leading point for an intussusception, thus creating an obstruction of the gut (see Case 12). Inflammation of the diverticulum can lead to signs and symptoms similar to those seen in appendicitis. Obstructive and inflammatory symptoms are more common in older children and adults.

The correct order in which to do GI studies—upper GI study, barium enema, endoscopy, Meckel's scan, etc.—should be at the discretion of the consultant. However, since Meckel's diverticulum is overall the most common cause of massive GI bleeding at this age, the decision was made in the emergency department to order a sodium pertechnetate Tc 99m scan first. The radioisotope is picked up by the parietal cells present in gastric mucosa (normal or ectopic). Older studies report a positive rate of 50%, but newer studies using careful patient preparation have improved the positive yield to between 90% and 98%. This child's scan was positive, and surgery was scheduled.

SUGGESTED READINGS

Cox K, Ament ME: Upper gastrointestinal bleeding in children and adolescents. *Pediatrics* 1979;63:408.

Farthing MG, et al: Occult bleeding from Meckel's diverticulum. *Br J Surg* 1981;68:176.

Macky WC, Dineen P: A fifty year experience with Meckel's diverticulum. *Surg Gynecol Obstet* 1983;156:56.

Sfakianakis GN, Conway JJ: Detection of ectopic gastric mucosa in Meckel's diverticulum and in other aberrations by scintigraphy: I. Pathophysiology and 10 year clinical experience. *J Nucl Med* 1981;22:647.

Sfakianakis GN, Conway JJ: Detection of ectopic gastric mucosa in Meckel's diverticulum and in other aberrations by scintigraphy: II. Indications and methods—A ten year experience. *J Nucl Med* 1981;22:732.

Physical Examination

HEENT: *Head*: closed fontanelles. *Eyes*: sunken; PERRLA; EOM intact; normal fundi; normal conjunctivae and sclerae; no tears. *Ears*: normal tympanic membranes. *Oropharynx*: mouth dry and parched; no visible pharyngitis or other enanthem

NECK: Supple; negative Kernig and Brudzinski signs; no stridor; no nodes; midline trachea

CHEST: Clear, although increased rate, without subcostal or intercostal retraction; no rales, rhonchi, or wheezing

ABD: Scaphoid; increased bowel sounds; no high-pitched tinkles or rushes; no organomegaly; no mass; no tenderness; no costovertebral angle tenderness; no palpable liver, kidneys, spleen

GU: *Rectum*: nontender; copious, foul-smelling, greenish mucoid diarrhea; heme + +

EXT: Decreased turgor; no clubbing, cyanosis, or edema

NEURO: Lethargic; irritable; very arousable; normoreflexive; normal motor-sensory examination; normal cranial nerve evaluation; no ataxia; no pathologic reflexes

SUGGESTED INTERVENTIONS

1. Administer oxygen, 4 L/min via nasal prongs.
2. Place on cardiac monitor.
3. Start IV with normal saline, bolus, 230 mL (i.e., 20 mL × 11.5 kg).
4. Remeasure vital signs, including posturals if normotensive; if still hypotensive, or pulse increases 10% going from supine to upright, rebolus as in No. 3; repeat until blood pressure normalizes to systolic of 80 to 85 mm Hg and no postural change.
5. Place urinary catheter to straight drainage; measure minute to minute volume; order urinalysis and culture and sensitivity on initial specimen.
6. Order blood chemistries/tests: Immediate Dextrostix® (if Dextrostix® value is less than 60 mg/dL, give 1 mL/kg 50% dextrose in water push and switch IV to 5% dextrose in normal saline); order CBC, blood culture, glucose, electrolytes, BUN, creatinine, and type and hold.
7. Order stool culture; stain for polymorphonuclear leukocytes, stool pH, and reducing substances.
8. Admit the patient.

CASE DISCUSSION

Diarrhea and dehydration is an extremely common problem in infants presenting to emergency departments for care. It is important for the emergency department physician to be comfortable with fluid and electrolyte management of these children. Underresuscitation and too aggressive overloading are equally undesirable. The underlying cause is secondary in importance to expedient accurate correction of deficits. However, initial studies are necessary to quantitate the degree of dehydration and depletion, as well as to determine the underlying disease. The physical presentation of the infant or child generally suggests the percentage of dehydration, according to the following paradigm:

	Total Body	Signs/Symptoms
Minimal Dehydration	5% loss	Loss of water (i.e., dry eyes, dry mouth, thirst); minimal tachycardia
Moderate Dehydration	10% loss	Structural changes: sunken fontanelle, sunken eyes, decreasing turgor; moderate tachycardia; postural hypotension; early acidosis
Severe Dehydration	15% loss	Systemic changes; gross hypotension; oliguria, anuria; poor skin perfusion; tachypnea; decreased level of consciousness; marked acidosis

These parameters, in general, are true for isotonic dehydration; however, one must note that in hypotonic (decreased serum sodium) dehydration, the signs and symptoms "lead" (i.e., appear at quantitatively lower levels of percentage weight loss) the degree of dehydration, whereas in hypertonic (increased serum sodium) dehydration the signs and symptoms "lag" the degree of percentage loss. This accounts for the frequency of underestimation of severity of the "hypertonics" and overestimation of the severity in the "hypotonics." Since the hypertonics are generally under 1 year of age, the serious mistakes are usually made in the evaluation of these latter, smaller, younger infants. As will be indicated later (see Case 18), the management of hypertonic dehydration is difficult and fraught with more serious complications than the other forms. So both diagnosis and treatment of hypertonic dehydration may present difficulties for the career emergency department physician who is not intimately experienced in pediatrics.

Hypotonic dehydration is characterized by solute loss in excess, proportionately, to the water loss. Examples are mineralocorticoid deficiency states, salt-losing nephropathy and enteropathy, cystic fibrosis, and excessive sweating. Another important etiology is inappropriate correction of losses with too dilute fluids.

In hypotonic dehydration the loss of external volume is compounded by an additional "loss" to the intracellular space in an attempt to achieve osmotic neutrality in the extracellular space. This "double" loss accounts for the exacerbation of signs and symptoms indicated above. These signs and symptoms are predominantly "extracellular" symptoms. Conversely, in hypertonic dehydration, although there are significant losses to the outside, there is a "contribution" to the extracellular space from the intracellular, once again to achieve osmotic neutrality, and this contribution tends to forestall the appearance of the true "extracellular" symptoms. However, this is at the expense of the intracellular space, so "intracellular" symptoms appear early and should be looked for: such symptoms are "doughy" skin, turgor, high-pitched irritable cry, and seizures. The common etiologies for hypertonic dehydration generally involve the loss of water in excess of solute, such as in diabetes insipidus (central or nephrogenic), glucocorticoid deficiency, excessive insensitive losses, and winter steam heating. Also, injudicious replacement of losses with too high tonic fluids will produce hypertonicity. There have been tragic accidents in the compounding of infant formulae, in which salt is accidentally replaced for sugar, resulting in disastrous hypertonicity. Feeding boiled skim milk formula is a well-recognized cause of hypertonicity.

This child, for whatever etiology, presented dehydrated 10% to 15% and was in shock. We like to use a rough approximate of normal systolic blood pressure equal to the weight (in kilograms) added to 70 mm Hg. Therefore, this 13-kg child should have had an estimated normal systolic blood pressure of 83 (80 to 85) mm Hg and was in fact about 10% below this. This approximation is only good for children over 1 year of age. For infants younger than 1 year of age, we use 60 mm Hg systolic as a minimum acceptable blood pressure. We favor Doppler-monitored blood pressure determination such as the Dynamapp® or Omega® for our infants and younger children.

The treatment of the hypotensive, dehydrated infant or child follows fairly specific guidelines. Start with only full tonic crystalloid normal saline; this will be perfectly appropriate for all the possibilities (i.e., hypotonic, isotonic, or hypertonic dehydration), so the emergency department physician does not have to agonize over choice of fluids—just start off with normal saline. Volume replacment *must* precede actual determination, via laboratory tests, of the actual type of dehydration. Over 15% reduction in expected systolic pressure and/or systemic manifestation of shock indicates rapid infusion of crystalloid until the blood pressure normalizes. The initial line must be that which can most readily be established. A second line is always indicated for persistent hypotension. The use of the MAST suit to reverse hypovolemic shock has been very well adapted to the pediatric patient. It also can make veins appear where they were absent prior to the inflation of the suit. We do not favor use of the abdominal compartment of the suit in nontraumatic forms of hypovolemic shock.

In less manifest cases of dehydration and hypotension (i.e., 10% or less by physical findings, 10% or less reduction of systolic pressure, or postural hypotension only), we favor the bolus approach to repletion, whereby normal saline is infused in rapid aliquots of 20 mL/kg and constant reappraisal of vital signs indicates when the aliquots may be discontinued, in favor of a more constant, calculated infusion rate.

As in all shock states, urine catheterization is used for initial urinalysis and culture, as well as continuous monitoring of urine output. We accept no less than 1 mL/kg/hr as a guideline for oliguria. After adequate volume loading (central venous pressure?), a dosage of furosemide (Lasix®) may be used if renal output is still below this parameter. We favor 1 mg/kg as the initial dosage of furosemide.

The actual determination of the type of dehydration depends on the laboratory studies that were sent off initially. Since this child was also febrile with heme + + stools and hypotensive, a CBC, blood culture, and type and hold were sent initially.

The electrolytes, BUN, and creatinine values all help to confirm the degree of dehydration, assess the tonicity of the dehydration, estimate the degree of acidosis, and finally indicate any potassium abnormalities. The cardiac monitor should always be checked initially for early clues on the tracing attributable to hypokalemia or hyperkalemia. The serum glucose level confirms the Dextrostix® determination. In this case the Dextrostix® was 80 to 100 mg/dL, so there was no need for glucose "push." It must be added that occasionally hypertonic dehydration is associated with hyperglycemia of moderate degree. This rarely needs insulin correction and disappears with amelioration of the hypovolemia and hypernatremia, but it would be unwise to use a dextrose solution on a child whose glucose level is already in the 200 to 400 mg/dL range. This once again underlines the importance of the Dextrostix® being done early in the evaluation. Also, in severe dehydration states in which the child has not been able to aliment from vomiting or toxicity, profound hypoglycemia may be present. Remember that the presentation of Addisonian crisis is hypovolemia, hypotension, and hypoglycemia.

Hypocalcemia is associated with hypertonic dehydration and once again rarely needs calcium infusion for correction but does need to be identified and followed. The Q_o-T_c interval* on the ECG can suggest hypocalcemia if it is prolonged. Very prolonged intervals, Chvostek's sign, or actual seizures would be indications for calcium infusion.

The chief complaint of this child was copious, protracted, fetid, mucus-laden diarrhea. The most likely diagnosis leading to this clinical dehydration and hypotension was dehydration secondary to invasive enterocolitis. Stool culture was appropriately sent off, and an examination for stool polymorphonuclear leukocytes was done. This test was returned positive, with many polymorphonuclear leukocytes seen per high-powered field (methylene blue preparation), and this confirmed our suspicion. The Hematest® positivity makes *Shigella, Salmonella,* enteroinvasive *Escherichia coli,* and *Campylobacter* good possibilities. Low stool pH and presence of reducing substances both suggest a lactase deficiency in the brush border of the gut, a phenomenon very characteristically induced by enteroinvasive bacteria and accounting for the exacerbation of the diarrhea by milk products. The patient in this case study had positive reducing substances and an acidic stool pH of 5.5.

---

*Q wave onset to T wave completion.

The infant recovered from the hypotension after an initial infusion of normal saline of 20 mL/kg. A good strategy would be to run the infusion at one and one-half to two times maintenance volume, leaving the initial normal saline hanging, until laboratory results are returned. Subsequent hypotensive episodes can then be quickly remedied as indicated above. The emergency department physician should be fairly comfortable in initiating fluid and electrolyte orders for the patient's admission. This could be delegated to the admitting pediatrician, but the pediatrician may not be immediately available. The guidelines below should allow the emergency department physician to initiate orders.

Maintenance volume for the pediatric age range is dictated by the rule "100–50–20":

Weight (kg)	24-Hour Maintenance Volume (water)	Example
0–10 kg	100 mL/kg	8 kg = 800 mL/24 hr
10–20 kg	1,000 mL + *50* mL/kg × (kg − 10)	14 kg = 1,000 + 50 × (14 − 10) = 1,000 + 50 × 4 = 1,200 mL/24 hr
> 20 kg	1,500 mL + *20* mL/kg × (kg − 20)	28 kg = 1,500 + 20 × (28 − 20) = 1,500 + 20 × 8 = 1,500 + 160 = 1,660 mL/24 hr

Maintenance Electrolytes:
Na^+ = 3 mEq/kg/day
K^+ = 2 mEq/kg/day
Cl^- = 2 mEq/kg/day

Replacement volumes and electrolytes depend on the percentage estimate of weight loss and the duration of dehydration, which in turn indicated the relative proportion of intracellular and extracellular losses. The following guidelines are very helpful in this determination:

Dehydration Duration	Relative Percentage of Losses Extracellular vs. Intracellular				
	EC		IC		
0–2 days	75%	+	25%	=	100%
2–7 days	60%	+	40%	=	100%
> 7 days	50%	+	50%	=	100%

Composition of Spaces	Extracellular	Intracellular
Sodium	135 mEq/L	
Potassium		160 mEq/L
Chloride	100 mEq/L	

Deficit calculations for sodium, and free water depend on the following parameters:

1. Sodium space = 60% total body weight (TBW)
2. Free water deficit = 4 mL/kg for every point decrease in serum sodium desired
3. Replacement and deficit chloride is always ⅔ of replacement and deficit sodium.

After volume resuscitation of this patient, the laboratory studies were returned as follows:

Serum glucose	= 90 mEq/L
Serum sodium	= 120 mEq/L
Serum potassium	= 4.6 mEq/L
Serum chloride	= 85 mEq/L
Serum bicarbonate	= 15 mEq/L
Blood urea nitrogen	= 38 mEq/L
Serum creatinine	= 1.4 mEq/L

The calculation for fluid and electrolyte orders for admission would obey the following reasoning: By the mother's weight observation, as well as clinical presentation, we estimate that this normally 13.2-kg child lost 13% and presented 4 pounds or 1.8 kg less at 11.4 kg. The dehydration had been going on for 3 days. The calculations for maintenance, replacement, and deficit fluid and electrolytes are shown in the following "scorecard":

	Water	Sodium	Potassium	Chloride
Maintenance:	1,000 + 50 × (13.2 − 10) 1,160 mL	3 × 13 = 39 mEq	2 × 13 = 26 mEq	2 × 13 = 26 mEq
Replacement:	1.8 kg = 1,800 cc			
Extracellular	0.6 × 1,800 = 1,080 mL	135 × 1.08 = 146 mEq		2/3 × 146 = 97 mEq

Intracellular	$0.4 \times 1,800$ $= 720$ mL		$160 \times 0.72 =$ 115 mEq (administer one half of calculated*) 57 mEq	
Deficits:		$13.2 \times 0.6 \times$ $(135 - 120) =$ 119 mEq		80 mEq
Totals: Less amount given in emergency department:	2,960 mL $- 230$ (NS)	304 mEq $- 35$	83 mEq	203 mEq $- 35$
Remainder: (Amount per liter used):	2,630 mL (1,000)	269 mEq (102)	83 mEq (31)	168 mEq (63)

*Rule of thumb.

The appropriate solution would therefore be 5% dextrose in ⅔ normal saline, with potassium chloride 30 mEq/L (withhold for anuria or known hyperkalemia).

A general rule of thumb states that for infusion rate in isotonic and hypotonic dehydration, run IV to replace one half of the daily amount in the first 8 hours and then the second half in the ensuing 16 hours. Therefore, IV orders would appear as follows: 5% dextrose in ⅔ normal saline and potassium chloride, 30 mEq/L, to run at 165 mL/hr (for first 8 hours).

The above calculations and guidelines apply for hypotonic and isotonic dehydration. Serum sodium values above 150 mEq/L define hypertonic dehydration, and the physician must follow separate instructions for safe smooth correction of the losses, as well as safe smooth (and not too rapid) lowering of the serum sodium level. This subject is covered in Case 18. The patient in this case study had his fluid levels managed exactly as indicated above and was kept on IV fluids for 1½ days, started on oral clear liquids, and advanced to a "BRAT" (bread, rice, apples, toast) diet. He was kept off milk products temporarily. His stool culture grew *Salmonella*, and he was placed on ampicillin. He was discharged after 4 days in the hospital with regular, formed stools and positive weight gain.

SUGGESTED READINGS

Barness LA: Fluid and electrolyte therapy. In Gellis SS, Kagan BM (eds): *Current Pediatric Therapy*, ed 12. Philadelphia, WB Saunders, 1986.

Hochman HI, Grodin MA, Crone RK: Dehydration. *Pediatr Clin North Am* 1979;26:803, 826.

Weil WB, Beilie MD (eds): *Fluid and Electrolyte Metabolism in Infants and Children*. New York, Grune & Stratton, 1977.

Case 16

Eighteen-month-old Male with Stridor and Cyanosis

CASE PRESENTATION

An 18-month-old male was rushed into the emergency department by his parents at 3:30 AM in mid November because he could not breathe. The child, who had been well except for a mild "cold," awakened at 3 AM with a loud barking cough and difficulty breathing. The parents scooped up the child and brought him to the hospital. In an attempt to calm the child his mother had offered him a bottle, but after a few sips the child refused further attempts to feed him.

The child's past medical history was uncomplicated. There were no prior respiratory problems. The pregnancy, labor, and delivery were all normal, and all the child's immunizations were current. There were no prior hospitalizations or surgeries. There were no allergies to foods or drugs.

Vital Signs

Because the child became extremely upset during attempts to assess vital signs the respiratory rate was counted visually.

HR: 180 beats/min
RR: 65 beats/min
T: 38°C (100.4°F)
BP: deferred
WT: 13 kg (estimated)

Physical Examination

GEN: The child on arrival was noted to be making loud stridorous sounds with inspiration and expiration. There was severe sternal retraction with each inspiration. When the child was approached by a nurse or physician, the child became agitated and the respiratory distress increased. The child was noted to have cyanosis of the lips and fingertips.

CHEST: There was loud stridor with each inspiration, which was heard best in the neck.

SUGGESTED INTERVENTIONS

1. Place child on mother's lap in a treatment room equipped for pediatric intubation and resuscitation.
2. Administer oxygen, 6 L/min, via mask held to the child's face by the mother.
3. Notify otolaryngologist.
4. Administer racemic epinephrine, 0.2 mL of 2.5% solution diluted 1:8 with water, via mask.
5. Prepare for intubation with No. 4.0 and No. 3.5 uncuffed endotracheal tubes. This is done while waiting for the racemic epinephrine to be administered.
6. Have anteroposterior and lateral neck x-rays done in the emergency department.
7. Administer dexamethasone (Decadron®), 6 mg (0.5 mg/kg) IM.
8. Admit the patient.

CASE DISCUSSION

Croup is the most prevalent cause of upper airway obstruction in children. The disease occurs chiefly in children 6 months to 2½ years of age.

There are three kinds of croup. Laryngotracheobronchitis is the most common. Spasmodic croup causes an occasional case, and bacterial tracheitis is very rare.

A variety of viruses cause laryngotracheobronchitis. The illness may be without prodrome or preceded by a few days of mild upper respiratory tract symptoms. In the usual case the child goes to bed without symptoms only to awaken with a barking cough and stridor. The degree of respiratory distress may be mild to very severe. If the child is old enough to talk, the voice is generally hoarse. Since the child does not have a sore throat, he will usually drink fluids. If a fever is present, it is usually low grade. The symptoms tend to improve as daytime approaches only to recur again the next night. This waxing and waning continues for 3 to 4 days, at which time the child is well again.

Spasmodic croup can be defined as recurrent croup. The etiology of these cases may be allergic. A child may have repeated bouts of spasmodic croup up through teen years. The individual episodes tend to be short, often lasting only one night.

Bacterial tracheitis is the result of bacterial suprainfection in cases of laryngotracheitis. Influenza A and parainfluenza viruses are the most likely to be associated with suprainfection. The entire trachea and often the larger bronchi are involved and filled with thick mucus and pus. The child is toxic and has a high fever.

Croup can usually be diagnosed easily by history. However, there are several important illnesses to consider in the differential diagnosis.

Epiglottitis, a bacterial infection of the epiglottis, principally affects children 2 to 5 years of age. As the epiglottis swells, it obstructs the hypopharynx, leading to complete obstruction in 12 to 18 hours. These children have substantial fevers and very sore throats, which results in drooling.

Retropharyngeal abscesses are most common before 5 years of age, with the peak below 1 year of age. This bacterial infection may spread from adjacent nodes in the pharynx. A foreign body lodged in the hypopharynx can also lead to abscess formation. The disease may begin as cervical adenitis or without prodrome. Although dysphagia and respiratory distress do occur, these are late signs. The only early signs may be fever and torticollis.

Respiratory distress caused by a foreign body usually presents with sudden onset of choking or vomiting during the daytime. Once a foreign body has passed the vocal cords it may lodge in a bronchus, causing hyperinflation or atelectasis and a chronic cough. Localized rather than general wheezing results if the foreign body allows some air to pass by it.

Asthma usually can be easily distinguished from croup and other causes of respiratory tract obstruction. The exception could be a child whose bronchospasm is so great that not enough air is passing to create wheezing. This is especially prominent in infants. Children without upper airway noises or stridor should be carefully auscultated for the presence of an occasional wheeze.

Very young infants may have respiratory tract obstruction from a long list of congenital malformations, which invariably present before 6 months of age. Tracheal malacia, laryngeal hemangiomas, and tracheal obstruction from aberrant vessels, tumors, or an enlarged thyroid are a few of the problems seen in very small children.

Most cases of croup spontaneously subside with exposure to cool air or steam vapor. Thus the trip to the hospital frequently cures the problem. Parents can be advised to take the child into a steamy bathroom if the croup recurs after leaving the emergency department. If the steam does not help, the child should be brought back to the hospital. Occasionally a child arrives in severe distress, such as the patient in this case study. In these cases the distinction between croup and epiglottitis is more difficult, but the treatment for each at this stage is the same. The child is left sitting in a quiet treatment room with the parents present. Oxygen is offered to, but not forced on, the child. Immediate preparations are made in case an artificial airway is required. The child is given racemic epinephrine, which will reverse croup but not epiglottitis. Children who have received racemic epinephrine should always be admitted because a rebound may occur up to 6 hours after the treatment. Repeated treatment with racemic epinephrine usually reverses the rebound. Racemic epinephrine has no documented detrimental effect on epiglottitis, retropharyngeal abscess, or inhalation of a foreign body.

During administration of the racemic epinephrine, preparations should be made for intubation in case the child's condition worsens. Choose an endotracheal tube one-half size smaller than normally used for that aged child. Failure of the racemic epinephrine to relieve severe obstruction requires intubation.

Anteroposterior and lateral films (upright) of the neck can be taken in the emergency department at any time that the child is stable. In croup, the anteroposterior film will show narrowing below the larynx so that the air column resembles a church steeple. In epiglottitis the lateral film will reveal swelling of the epiglottis, which often resembles an ant hill. Radiopaque foreign bodies and retropharyngeal abscess can be diagnosed similarly.

In cases that are not severe enough for treatment with racemic epinephrine, the decision to admit should be made if the child has retractions and loud stridor at rest. Since croup tends to improve after the third day, the decision to admit can also be partially guided by the length of time the child has been ill.

Dexamethasone (Decadron®) has been shown to decrease the number of hospital days needed for resolution of croup symptoms and to improve the patient's subjective symptoms.

SUGGESTED READINGS

Currarino G, Williams B: Lateral inspiration and expiration radiographs of the neck in children with laryngotracheitis (croup). *Radiology* 1982;145:365.

Denny FW, Murphy TF, Clyde WA, et al: Croup: An 11 year study in a pediatric practice. *Pediatrics* 1983;71:871.

Fogel JM, Berg IJ, Gerber MA, et al: Racemic epinephrine in the treatment of croup: Nebulization alone versus nebulization with intermittent positive pressure breathing. *J Pediatr* 1982;101:1028.

Glezen WP, Loda FA, Clyde WA, et al: Epidemiology of acute lower respiratory disease of children in a pediatric practice. *J Pediatr* 1971;78:397.

Koren G, Frand M, Barzilay Z, et al: Corticosteroid treatment of laryngotracheitis v. spasmodic croup in children. *Am J Dis Child* 1983;137:941.

Liston SL, Gehrz RC, Siegel LG, et al: Bacterial tracheitis. *Am J Dis Child* 1983;137:764.

Singer OP, Wilson WJ: Laryngotracheitis: 2 years experience with racemic epinephrine. *Can Med Assoc J* 1976;115:132.

Case 17

Eighteen-month-old Male with Cough, Fever, Tachypnea, and Pallor

CASE PRESENTATION

An 18-month-old black male with known sickle cell disease (SS) presented with a 2-day history of fever, cough, and runny nose. He was feeding well until the day of presentation when he vomited once and refused all further fluids. His mother has noted an increased respiratory rate for 1 day. She denies any extremity pain or swelling. He has had a pneumococcal polysaccharide immunization at age 1 year but is not on prophylactic antibiotics. His usual medications include folic acid and vitamins. He was admitted 3 months ago with pneumonia during a crisis. She gave him acetaminophen about 12 hours ago.

Vital Signs

BP: 90/60 mm Hg
HR: 120 beats/min
RR: 45/min
T: 39.8°C (103.6°F)
WT: 12 kg

Physical Examination

GEN: Alert male in mild respiratory distress, playing with a set of keys
HEENT: *Head:* NCAT. *Eyes:* icteric sclerae; clear conjunctivae; EOM intact; PERRLA; flat discs. *Ears:* normal tympanic membranes. *Nose:* nares have a clear discharge. *Oropharynx:* no injection; enlarged tonsils

NECK: Supple with nontender shotty cervical adenopathy; negative Kernig and Brudzinski signs

CHEST: Mild intercostal retractions; rales in right base with no dullness

CVS: Tachycardia without S_3 or S_4; grade II/VI systolic ejection murmur at the left upper sternal border; normal pulses

ABD: Normoactive bowel sounds; no tenderness or masses; spleen tip palpable; liver 2 cm below right costal margin

GU: Normal male with no priapism

EXT: No swelling, erythema, or tenderness; no cyanosis

NEURO: Alert; cranial nerves intact; reflexes, motor and sensory responses, and coordination normal

SKIN: No cyanosis

SUGGESTED INTERVENTIONS

1. Administer acetaminophen, 120 mg PO (10 mg/kg).
2. Administer oxygen, 5 L/min via mask.
3. Order blood specimens for CBC, reticulocyte count, blood culture and sensitivity, type and hold, ABGs.
4. Order portable chest x-ray.
5. Perform urinalysis.
6. Establish an IV line and give 5% dextrose in ¼ normal saline to run at 80 mL/hr (1½ to 2 times normal maintenance):

$$\text{Maintenance} = 100 \text{ mL/kg} \times d = 1200 \text{ mL/24 hr} = 50 \text{ mL/hr}$$

7. Order ampicillin, 450 mg IV every 6 hours (150 mg/kg/day). Give initial 50 mg/kg IVSD in emergency department.
8. Admit patient for hydration, IV antibiotics therapy, and observation.

CASE DISCUSSION

Bacterial infection is a major threat to young children with sickle cell disease. As many as 30% of all deaths among individuals with sickle cell anemia occur before the age of 5 years. The majority of these deaths are caused by bacterial infection with encapsulated organisms. Individuals with sickle cell disease are predisposed to infection because of their relative immunologic incompetence with abnormal opsonization, phagocytosis, complement activation, and functional asplenia. The incidence of unsuspected bacteremia in hematologically normal children under 2 years of age with fever is reported as 2% to 4%. In children with sickle cell disease and fever the incidence increases to 10% to 30%. Among healthy children the outcome of occult bacteremia with pneumococcus regardless of therapy has been good. When the offending organism is *Hemophilus influenzae* the results have not been as favorable, with an increased incidence of focal infections. In children with sickle cell disease the outcome of bacteremia with pneumococcus and *H. influenzae* is much more alarming, with serious infection occurring in up to 50% of bacteremic patients. In order to avoid unnecessary morbidity and mortality the physician needs to have an increased awareness of those children likely to be bacteremic.

The search for the patient who is bacteremic begins with the initial examination. The most predictive and sensitive clinical indicators of bacteremia are eye movements and motor functions. These include such observations as whether the child will regard the mother's or examiner's face and whether the child will reach for objects and engage in play. Based on these observations, reports indicate a 70% sensitivity in detecting bacteremic children. The most common presentation of bacteremic children with sickle cell disease is a fever without any identifiable source; however, there is a remarkable diversity of presentation. In one series, while 41% had the often-described acute onset of fever and few associated symptoms, 59% had a more gradual prodromal illness of 1 to 7 days' duration. The symptoms most commonly encountered in the prodrome of children with sickle cell disease and proven sepsis are lethargy, GI symptoms such as vomiting, and extremity pain. Although pneumonia accounts for the majority of hospital admissions for infection in children with sickle cell disease, they are more prone to meningitis, septic arthritis, osteomyelitis, and urinary tract infections than their hematologically normal counterparts. There does not appear to be supporting evidence for the claim that infections predispose to crisis. However, there is evidence that the presence of concurrent infection and crisis has a higher mortality rate.

In hematologically normal children under 2 years of age, a temperature greater than 38.9°C (102.0°F), WBC count greater than 15,000/cu mm, and polymorphic band counts over 1,000/cu mm are predictive of bacteremias. Five percent of patients fulfilling these criteria have a positive blood culture, and 70% of patients with a positive blood culture fulfill these criteria. In children with sickle cell disease the findings are less reliable, although a WBC count greater than 20,000/cu mm and a temperature greater than 40°C (104°F) are significantly associated with bacteremia. The workup of a febrile child with sickle cell disease should include a CBC, reticulocyte count, blood culture, and urinalysis. The hemoglobin and reticulocyte values can be compared with previous values for the individual to aid in the diagnosis of aplastic, sequestration, and hemolytic crises. A chest x-ray may be positive for infiltrate even if there is a paucity of auscultatory findings. In children, especially if they are dehydrated, rales may only be heard after several hours of rehydration. Additional studies such as a lumbar puncture, arthrocentesis, blood gas analysis, and bone scan may be needed depending on the presentation of the patient. Determination of the ESR in patients with sickle cell disease is not helpful since it is usually low. The evaluation of a febrile child at risk for sickle cell disease should include a standard solubility test and hemoglobin electrophoresis.

Streptococcus pneumoniae and *H. influenzae* are the most common pathogens of sepsis and meningitis. However, enteric organisms such as *Salmonella* are also occurring with increased frequency. The risk for pneumococcal infection is increased 400-fold and *H. influenzae* infection 4-fold in children with sickle cell disease compared with hematologically normal children.

Since no single physical finding or laboratory test can accurately identify the septic patient, most centers hospitalize and begin IV antibiotic therapy in febrile patients with sickle cell disease who are under 4 to 5 years of age. For any child with sickle cell disease and fever managed as an outpatient, reevaluation is mandatory within 24 hours.

Antibiotic therapy to cover *S. pneumoniae* and *H. influenzae* usually consists of ampicillin or the combination of ampicillin and chloramphenicol in children who appear toxic. Most centers are reporting about a 20% resistance rate of *H. influenzae* to ampicillin. Antibiotic therapy needs to be continually reevaluated depending on culture results and clinical course. In patients with sickle cell disease and pneumococcal sepsis, there is a high reported rate of complications, including disseminated intravascular coagulation and cardiovascular collapse, associated with adrenal hemorrhagic necrosis. At the first sign of cardiovascular impairment, stress doses of corticosteroids (e.g., methylprednisolone sodium succinate [Solu-Medrol®], 2 mg/kg, IVp) should be administered. To prevent dehydration and vaso-occlusive crises, hydration should be maintained at one and one-half to two times normal. Administration of oxygen is indicated to prevent hypoxia and further sickling. Analgesia should be provided if there is any report of pain with the choice aided by the individual's previous record.

Pneumococcal polysaccharide immunization has been documented to increase opsonic activity and antibody formation in individuals with sickle cell disease, but the response is unreliable in children under 2 years of age. Because of the systemic involvement and psychological support required by individuals with sickle cell disease, primary care through an emergency department should be discouraged, and all patients should be referred to a hematologist or physician familiar with sickle cell disease for long-term follow-up.

SUGGESTED READINGS

Barret-Connor E: Bacterial infection and sickle cell anemia. *Medicine* 1971;50:97.

Bratton L, Teele DW, Klein JO, et al: Outcome of unsuspected pneumococcemia in children not initially admitted to the hospital. *J Pediatr* 1977;90:703.

Chudwin DS, Wara DW, Matthay KK, et al: Increased serum opsonic activity and antibody concentration in patients with sickle cell disease after pneumococcal polysaccharide immunization. *J Pediatr* 1983;102:51.

Kravis E, Fleisler G, Ludwig S, et al: Fever in children with sickle cell hemoglobinopathies. *Am J Dis Child* 1982;136:1075.

McCarthy PL, Jekel J, Stashwick C, et al: Further definition of history and observation variables in assessing febrile children. *Pediatrics* 1981;67:687.

McIntosh S, Rooks Y, Ritchey AK, et al: Fever in young children with sickle cell disease. *J Pediatr* 1980;96:199.

Nottidge V: Pneumococcal meningitis in sickle cell disease in childhood. *Am J Dis Child* 1983;137:29.

Powars D, Overturf G, Turner E: Natural history of sickle cell disease—the first ten years. *Semin Hematol* 1975;12:257.

Powars D, et al: Is there an increased risk of *Hemophilus influenzae* septicemia in children with sickle cell anemia. *Pediatrics* 1983;71:927.

Teele D, Pelton SI, Grant MJ, et al: Bacteremia in febrile children under 2 years of age: Results of cultures of blood of 600 consecutive febrile children seen in a walk-in clinic. *J Pediatr* 1975;87:227.

Thirteen-month-old Female with Diarrhea, Weight Loss, and Irritable High-pitched Cry

CASE PRESENTATION

A 13-month-old black female presented to the emergency department with a 4-day history of diarrhea, refusal to feed, low-grade temperature, and irritability and a high-pitched cry. She had had some respiratory congestion prior to the onset of the diarrhea, unassociated with fever. Her stools became soft; then diarrhea occurred on the fourth day prior to presentation. Her normal weight was 26 pounds according to the mother, and she was now down to about 23 pounds. Her diarrhea was described as loose brown, no mucus, no blood, and not particularly malodorous. She then began to refuse solids and was being maintained on clear liquids. On the day of presentation the mother noted increased irritability and the onset of a high-pitched cry. The mother noted sunken eyeballs and a low-grade temperature (100°F rectal).

The child had a negative past medical history, had had a normal pregnancy and delivery, and left the hospital on the day of delivery, with no perinatal jaundice, fever, or respiratory problems. Her growth and development were all normal, all immunizations were current, and there was a negative family history for sickle cell disease.

Vital Signs

T: 38.4°C (101.1°F, rectal)
P: 180 beats/min
BP: 60 mm hg (palpable)
RR: 25/min
WT: 10.7 kg

Physical Examination

HEENT: *Head:* anterior fontanelle slightly open and flat. *Eyes:* PERRLA; EOM intact; normal fundi; absent tears; normal conjunctivae and sclerae. *Ears:* normal tympanic membranes. *Oropharynx:* dry mouth; no exanthem; no acetone on breath

NECK: Supple; negative Kernig and Brudzinski signs; no nodes; normal trachea; no stridor

CHEST: Clear to percussion and auscultation; rate increases; no rales, rhonchi, wheezing, or retractions; nontender to palpation

CVS: Normal S_1, S_2, P_2; no murmurs, gallop rhythms, rubs, or lifts; point of maximal impulse normally placed

ABD: Soft; scaphoid; normal bowel sounds; no masses; no rebound; no palpable liver, spleen, kidneys; costovertebral angle tenderness; no bruises

GU: Loose, brown stools; heme −; stool negative for polymorphonuclear leukocytes and reducing substances; pH normal

EXT: No cyanosis, clubbing, or edema; nontender; moved all extremities well

NEURO: Lethargic, but arousable; irritable cry; nonconsolable; good eye contact and body movement; normoreflexive; no ataxia; no pathologic reflexes; responds to pain appropriately; follows simple commands; responds to name

SKIN: No exanthem; slightly "doughy" consistency with decreased turgor; no bruises

SUGGESTED INTERVENTIONS

1. Administer oxygen, 3 L/min, via nasal prongs.
2. Place on cardiac monitor.
3. Start IV with normal saline, rapid infusion 215 mL (20 mL/kg). Reassess postural vital signs.
4. Order blood specimens for Dextrostix®, CBC, blood culture, ESR, electrolytes, BUN, creatinine, glucose, toxicologic screen, liver function tests, ammonia, acetone, sickle prep.
5. Perform urinalysis, urine culture and sensitivity, and test for urine sugar and acetone.
6. Give ampicillin 535 mg (50 mg/kg) IVSD, and chloramphenicol 265 mg (25 mg/kg) IVSD.
7. Order stool culture.
8. Order chest x-ray (portable).

9. Order CT scan.
10. Order lumbar puncture.
11. Admit the patient.

CASE DISCUSSION

The emergency department physician was confronted with a perplexing problem of a 13-month-old infant with an abnormal level of consciousness described as irritable, lethargic, and nonconsolable. The child had a low-grade temperature and had 3 to 4 days of loose stools and diarrhea, following an upper respiratory tract type prodrome. There was no history of trauma, intoxicants, and infectious diseases in the family and no prior history suggestive of gradual deterioration, loss of developmental milestones, and seizures.

The physician appropriately followed a differential diagnosis including infectious, metabolic, toxicologic, traumatic, and encephalopathic etiologies. But first he addressed the most immediate problem—the patient's hypotension. The child had a 10% documented weight loss according to the mother's observation. The "bolus" method of repletion was used, giving 20 mL/kg in rapid fashion, using full-strength crystalloid, normal saline. The Dextrostix® initially was modestly elevated, so no glucose was included in the infusion. The diagnosis of diabetic ketoacidosis was entertained and appropriate laboratory studies were sent off. This proved negative. Oxygen therapy and routine cardiac monitoring were instituted. Basic laboratory studies looking for clues to the list of etiologies were ordered. Toxicologic causes for decreased level of consciousness are very common in pediatrics and must always be remembered by the emergency department physician. Nothing on physical examination suggested trauma or child abuse, but this is another area that has high yield in the differential of decreased level of consciousness. The CT scan was obtained to rule out cerebral trauma, as well as other lesions (tumor, abscess, hemorrhage) that could have presented in this manner. In the nonmeningismic patient who is neither toxic nor grossly febrile, it is important to rule out a mass lesion first by way of the cerebral CT scan, then complete the evaluation with the lumbar puncture, looking for infectious/inflammatory etiologies for the neurologic status. In difficult cases when there is strong suspicion of both etiologies, pushing appropriate antibiotics is recommended first, then performing the CT scan as rapidly as possible, and, if negative, following through with the lumbar puncture. In this case the CT scan, done first, was negative, and subsequent lumbar puncture proved negative.

The laboratory studies were returned immediately after the patient had the lumbar puncture:

CBC: Hemoglobin/hematocrit: 11.4 mg/dL/34%
              WBC: 7,800/cu mm
              Differential: 65 segments, 5 bands, 20 lymphocytes, 5 mono-
              cytes, 1 basophil, 4 eosinophils.
              Platelets: normal
Electrolytes: Sodium: 170 mEq/L
              Potassium: 4.3 mEq/L
              Chloride: 125 mEq/L
              Bicarbonate: 15 mEq/L
BUN: 45 mg/dL
Creatinine: 1.3 mg/dL
Glucose: 255 mg/dL
Calcium: 4.3 mg/dL (ionized)
Ammonia and liver function tests: normal

This child represented a fairly classic presentation of hypernatremic dehydra-tion, with irritability, lethargy, high-pitched cry, doughy skin, and a course of 3 to 4 days. The urine was appropriately concentrated, making diabetes insipidus unlikely, and the urine similarly was not infected.

The emergency department fluid and electrolyte repletion orders must be designed to accomplish two goals: (1) to reverse immediately any hypotension and (2) to complete the sodium correction slowly so that the serum osmolarity is not dropped too fast, a situation that exposes the hypertonic brain to too much free water, potentially causing cerebral edema, seizure, and death. This complication occurs more frequently in developed countries using sophisticated IV techniques than in underdeveloped countries, where economics prohibit parenteral therapy. There is a lesson to be learned from this experience, and it translates into the dictum of "go slow!" The "scorecard" that was developed for the calculation of fluid and electrolytes will be reviewed for this hypertonically dehydrated child (as in Case 15).

A very important guideline to safe replacement is to plan a daily reduction in serum sodium no more than 15 points *or* one half the amount from initial sodium to a desired sodium of 135 mEq/L, whichever is least! For example, in this case the serum sodium value starts out at 170 mEq/L, and the desired value is 135 mEq/L. Thus there is a difference of 25 points, half of which would be 12.5 points (use 13). This is less than 15 points, and therefore the goal for the first day's reduction will be 13 points reduction in the serum sodium level. Administer 4 mL/kg/day free water to achieve one point reduction in serum sodium. This means that this child will receive 4 × 13 (points) × 10.7 (kg) = 556 mL of "deficit" free water in the first day. Analogous to deficit sodium in Case 15, deficit free water will show up in the scorecard in this case of hypernatremic dehydration.

Actual patient weight: 10.7 kg
Desired patient weight: 11.8 kg
Percent of dehydration: 10%
Serum sodium: 170 mEq/L
Days of dehydration: 3
Initial bolus: 215 mL normal saline

	Water	*Sodium*	*Potassium*	*Chloride*
Maintenance:	1090 mL	36 mEq	24 mEq	24 mEq
Replace:	1180 mL (10% of 11.8 kg)			
	Extracellular (%60) 700 mL	95 mEq		63 mEq
	Intracellular (%40) 480 mL		38 mEq 76 mEq calculated; administer ½ calculated*	
Deficits:	free water 556			
Totals:	2,826 mL	131 mEq	62 mEq	87 mEq
Less Push:	215 mL	33 mEq		33 mEq
Net Result:	2,611 mL	98 mEq	62 mEq	54 mEq
(Amounts per liter used):	(1,000)	(38)	(24)	(20)

*Rule of thumb.

Since this solution approximates 0.25 normal saline, it is too dilute to start off replacement for hypertonic dehydration. If calculated tonicity is less than 0.5 normal saline, use 0.5 normal saline as the initial fluid. This is a safety factor, designed to prevent too rapid drop in the serum sodium value. Also, contrary to the rate guideline in Case 15, hypertonic dehydration is replaced smoothly, with no increment for the first 8 hours; instead, the desired amount is given evenly over the entire 24 hours. Potassium is held for oliguria/anuria or known hyperkalemia. Most children with diarrhea are total body potassium depleted, so serum potassium is carefully monitored during the course of repletion. Since the initial glucose level was high, 5% dextrose can be withheld until Dextrostix® falls to 100 to 150 mg/dL. Therefore, infusion will be 0.5 normal saline at 110 mL/hr = 2,611 mL/24 hr. Each liter will contain 24 mEq potassium chloride.

All other diagnostic studies were normal, with no indication of bacterial infection. All cultures of blood, CSF, urine, and stool were negative, but a stool Rotazyme® study done as an inpatient was positive. The toxicologic screen was similarly negative.

This child had an uncomplicated resolution of her viral enteritis and of her hypernatremia and was off parenteral therapy by the third day with adequate weight gain.

SUGGESTED READINGS

Please see Case 15.

Eighteen-month-old Male with Irritability and Cyanosis

CASE PRESENTATION

An 18-month-old, 9.5-kg, white male was noted to be cyanotic at birth and was diagnosed as having tetralogy of Fallot at catheterization and angiography at 4 days of age. He has been small for age and occasionally cyanotic with crying but otherwise has had no problems since the neonatal period. He is followed by a cardiologist and is taking no medications.

The infant was well until this morning when he awoke and had a cyanotic spell while eating breakfast. His mother noted that he began crying during his meal and became progressively cyanotic. Within 15 minutes he began to breathe deeply and rapidly and became a pale blue color. On the way to the hospital he has been fretful and irritable and appears increasingly lethargic.

There has been no history of fever or other signs of systemic illness.

Vital Signs

T: 38.6°C (101.5°F)
P: 160 beats/min
RR: 65/min
BP: 90/50 mm Hg

Physical Examination

GEN: Small, pale, cyanotic infant who is tachypneic and hyperpneic, alert, but fretful and irritable and who when left alone would assume a crouched prone position with his legs tucked under the abdomen

HEENT: Significant for cyanotic mucous membranes and scattered petechiae on the face
NECK: No distention of neck veins
CHEST: No rales, rhonchi, or wheezes; prominent subcostal and intercostal retractions; accessory muscles used in respiration
CVS: Hyperactive precordium with heave along the left sternal border; no thrills; S_1 normal; S_2 loud and single; grade III/VI systolic ejection-quality murmur at upper left sternal border; no diastolic or to–fro murmur; no gallop rhythm
ABD: Soft with no organomegaly
EXT: Weak, but palpable and symmetric pulses in all extremities; capillary refill delayed at 2 to 3 seconds; no edema; 2+ clubbing
NEURO: Alert, oriented, crying, irritable; moves all extremities well; normal motor-sensory examination; no ataxia; normoreflexive

SUGGESTED INTERVENTIONS

1. Administer oxygen, 3 to 4 L/min, via mask or nasal cannula.
2. Place lead II ECG monitoring electrodes.
3. Give morphine sulfate, 0.2 mg/kg SC.
4. Establish IV access—5% dextrose in water, KVO.
5. Order blood specimens for ABGs, CBC, Dextrostix®, and blood group type; hold clot for cross-match.
6. Place child in knee-chest position (as he is doing himself).
7. Allow 15 to 20 minutes for improvement if patient is stable.
8. If no improvement, treat metabolic acidosis with sodium bicarbonate; should patient be digitalized, assure normokalemia or hyperkalemia prior to giving a bolus of bicarbonate: 1 to 2 mEq/kg/dose depending on the severity of base deficit.
9. If hematocrit is not appropriate for degree of cyanosis (45% to 60%), have blood cross-matched for transfusion. If hematocrit is greater than 65% to 70%, infuse fresh frozen plasma or 5% human serum albumin at 5 mL/kg over 20 to 30 minutes; *do not* phlebotomize.
10. If no improvement, consider propranolol, 0.02 mg/kg, every 10 to 15 minutes to maximum of 0.1 mg/kg.
11. Admit patient to cardiology service.

CASE DISCUSSION

In the patient in this case, the ABG analysis showed a pH of 7.20, $Paco_2$, 22 mm Hg; Pao_2, 20 mm Hg; HCO_3^-, 8 mEq/L; and base excess, −15. The hemoglobin/hematocrit was 12.6 g/dL/38% with a mean corpuscular volume of 79. Dextrostix® was 80 to 100 mg/dL. The patient successfully improved with morphine, 0.2 mg/kg SC, and sodium bicarbonate, 4 mEq/kg, in three divided doses. Two hours later his ABG was pH, 7.35; $Paco_2$, 40 mm Hg; Pao_2, 45 mm Hg; HCO_3^-, 22 mEq/L; and base excess, -1.3. He was transfused with 5 mL/kg of packed RBCs. After this acute admission he was sent home on propranolol and ferrous sulfate and was eventually operated on at 2 years of age after two additional severe hypoxic ("TET") spells.

Tetralogy of Fallot accounts for only about 10% of all congenital heart disease but it is the most common diagnosis in cyanotic patients older than 1 year of age. It is approximately equal in incidence in males and females and carries no specific correlation to a syndrome or genetic condition.

The four defects that make up the "tetralogy" are ventricular septal defect, dextroposition of the aortic root, right ventricular hypertrophy, and pulmonary outflow tract obstruction, which may be manifest as narrowing of the pulmonary artery or its branches, the pulmonary valve, the annulus, or the muscular infundibulum. All patients with tetralogy of Fallot have some infundibular hypertrophy, however. The degree of compromise is related to the magnitude of the gradient across the right ventricular outflow tract, which leads to a right-to-left shunt across the ventricular septal defect, which is usually large and therefore unrestrictive.

Tetralogy of Fallot is complicated by paroxysms of cyanosis and respiratory distress termed *cyanotic spells, hypoxemic spells,* or *TET spells.* These consist of severe hypoxemia with resultant tissue hypoxia and acidosis, accompanied by hyperpnea and tachypnea. In the absence of intervention, they can resolve spontaneously or progress to severe acidosis, obtundation, and death. The spells typically occur in the morning, or after a nap, and are precipitated by a Valsalva maneuver, such as crying, defecation, or feeding.

The pathophysiology of these episodes is debatable; there are two major hypotheses. The first centers around a hyperpnea that develops as a response to tissue hypoxia secondary to increased metabolic demands following a period of inactivity (as in rising from a nap).

Hyperpnea causes an increase in negative intrathoracic pressure that normally leads to increased venous return, and increase in venous return leads to an increase in right-to-left shunting in those patients and worsening hypoxia. The hypoxia and acidosis cause an increase in pulmonary vascular resistance, leading to increased shunting and creating a "vicious cycle."

The second theory centers on worsening of the right ventricular outflow tract obstruction (frequently termed *spasm,* although cardiac muscle does not undergo tetany) secondary to tachycardia with decreased right ventricular end-diastolic volume, decreased venous return, and increased inotropy.

The modalities commonly used to treat a cyanotic spell can be seen to have a logical mechanism of action in either physiologic paradigm. Oxygen decreased the pulmonary vascular resistance and the stimulus to hyperpnea.

The knee–chest position (or squatting, as is sometimes seen spontaneously in these patients) has been said to increase venous return and alleviate right ventricular outflow tract obstruction. Some studies have refuted this, demonstrating an actual decrease in venous return. Squatting may work secondary to increasing systemic vascular resistance and lessening the right versus left resistance difference.

Morphine decreases pulmonary vascular resistance and inhibits the respiratory centers centrally. It was previously thought to block catecholamine-induced inotropism and thereby lessen contractility, but this has been disproven.

Sodium bicarbonate should be given to correct acidosis, since this, too, will lessen pulmonary vascular resistance, as well as decrease the respiratory drive to hyperpnea.

Propranolol decreases contractility, which may lessen right ventricular outflow tract obstruction, although its efficacy in pulmonary atresia suggests an additional mechanism. Propranolol also is a negative chronotropic agent, allowing for increased diastolic filling time. It blocks the decrease in systemic vascular resistance that follows acidosis. It also works centrally to block tachypnea triggered by hypoxemia. Propranolol is most commonly used orally to "prophylax" against further hypoxic spells. It is also effective intravenously to abort an ongoing attack, although a patient who has not responded to earlier methods should be admitted and this modality used on an inpatient basis. The oral dosage is 0.25 to 1.0 mg/kg every 6 hours.

Anemia can exacerbate hypoxic spells in that a decreased oxygen-carrying capacity increases tissue hypoxia and acidosis. Hematocrits less than 45% should be considered anemic in cyanotic congenital heart disease, especially if a mild-to-moderate microcytosis is found.

Spells that remain refractory after correction of hematologic and metabolic derangements and medical treatment can sometimes be aborted with general anesthesia, the mechanism of action of which is interruption of the hyperpnea–acidosis cycle.

Any patient with a cyanotic spell that requires treatment with medication should be admitted for observation and evaluation to be sure an underlying condition has not precipitated the spell.

SUGGESTED READINGS

Guntherroth WG, et al: Tetralogy of Fallot. In Adams FH (ed): *Moss' Heart Disease in Infants, Children, and Adolescents*, ed 3. Baltimore, Williams & Wilkins, 1983.

Morgan BC, et al: A clinical profile of paroxysmal hyperpnea in cyanotic congenital heart disease. *Circulation* 1965;31:66.

Nineteen-month-old Male with Fever, Vomiting, Diarrhea, and Irritability

CASE PRESENTATION

A normally 25-lb (11.5 kg) 19-month-old black male presented to the emergency department with a chief complaint of vomiting and diarrhea for 2 days. The patient's parents gave a history of upper respiratory tract symptoms for 2 weeks prior to presentation. Fever to 39.4°C (103°F) and two loose stools developed 2 days prior to admission, along with irritability, unsteady gait, and increased sleepiness. The patient was seen at another emergency department 1 day prior to admission and received treatment consisting of penicillin intramuscularly and an antiemetic. The patient remained febrile and on the morning of presentation he vomited once and appeared sleepy and lethargic. Past medical history was completely benign with normal pregnancy, labor, and delivery. Immunizations are all current. There were no prior hospitalizations or illnesses. The family history is negative for sickle cell anemia.

On presentation to the emergency department the patient was a robust 19-month-old who appeared mildly dehydrated. He lay on his back motionless and cried out irritably when moved about or examined. When placed in a sitting position, he maintained his balance but held his head in an opisthotonic fashion.

Vital Signs

BP: 90/60 mm Hg
HR: 140 beats/min
RR: 40/min
T: 39.2°C (102.6°F)
WT: 10.9 kg

Physical Examination

HEENT: *Head:* fontanelles closed. *Eyes:* PERRLA; fundi benign with flat discs. *Ears:* tympanic membranes red with abnormal landmarks, move well. *Oropharynx:* mucous membranes slightly dry; throat clear

NECK: Held in opisthotonic position; Brudzinski sign present; Kernig sign absent; shotty cervical adenopathy

CHEST: Clear to auscultation; no retractions

CVS: Grade II/VI systolic murmur at upper left sternal border; regular rate and rhythm; no gallop rhythm or rub

ABD: Soft; nontender; no organomegaly; normal bowel sounds

EXT: Good perfusion; pulses symmetric

NEURO: Lethargic but responds verbally to verbal stimuli; cranial nerves intact; no focal findings on examination of motor system and deep tendon reflexes

SKIN: No rash; normal turgor

SUGGESTED INTERVENTIONS

1. Obtain blood specimens for CBC, blood culture, glucose, electrolytes, BUN, creatinine, sickle preparation, and Dextrostix® (result = 90–120 mg/dL).
2. Establish IV access and begin maintenance hydration at 1,050 mL/day (45 mL/hr) with 5% dextrose in 0.25 normal saline.
3. Perform lumbar puncture. Send CSF for Gram stain, culture and sensitivity, cell count, protein, and glucose; include latex fixation or counterimmunoelectrophoresis for *Hemophilus influenzae.*

   a. If CSF is clear, await cell count and other data.
   b. If CSF is turbid or purulent do not wait, give ampicillin, 50 mg/kg IVSD, and 30 minutes later give chloramphenicol, 25 mg/kg IVSD, 15 minutes prior to analysis of any laboratory results.

4. Order urinalysis and urine culture and sensitivity.
5. Send stool for culture and Wright's stain for leukocytes.
6. Admit the patient and arrange for respiratory isolation.

CASE DISCUSSION

This patient's lumbar puncture showed 5,750 WBCs, 77% segments, 11% bands, 7% lymphocytes, 4% monocytes; protein, 206 mg/dL; glucose, 17 mg/dL.

Gram stain showed polymorphonuclear leukocytes and gram-negative pleomorphic rods. Latex fixation for *H. influenzae* was positive.

This case presented an interesting and fairly common diagnostic dilemma—the febrile child under 2 years of age with associated symptoms. Because he presented in winter, during the height of an epidemic of viral gastroenteritis, the patient was initially diagnosed as having this infection when he presented with fever, vomiting, and diarrhea. Several clues led to the increased suspicion for meningitis: the patient's posture and avoidance of motion or eye contact seemed out of proportion to his history of one or two loose stools, and his physical findings were consistent with only very mild dehydration (approximately 5%). Meningismus was present, as was Brudzinski sign.

The clinical diagnosis of meningitis in infants is frequently not straightforward. The history includes fever, lethargy, crying, vomiting, irritability increasing rather than decreasing when the child is held, and increased sleepiness or lethargy.

Physical findings of meningismus are not reliably present until 18 months of age, and the absence of meningismus should not be used to rule out the diagnosis prior to 2 years of age. Any child under 2 who presents with fever and has no obvious source (otitis media, purulent pharyngitis, upper respiratory tract symptoms) is a candidate for lumbar puncture. The presence of upper respiratory tract symptoms or diarrhea should not be sufficient to discourage the physician from performing a lumbar puncture in a patient who appears listless or hyperirritable. Published studies have shown absence of playfulness, "social" smile, and eye contact to be important in identifying children with sepsis and meningitis, but the use of these symptoms depends on the level of experience of the examiner in evaluating children.

Interpretation of lumbar puncture results can be complicated by the history of prior administration of antibiotics. The WBC count of the CSF is usually in the thousands with polymorphonuclear leukocytes predominant in patients with bacterial meningitis. The protein value is usually greater than 100 mg/dL, and the glucose level is less than 40 mg/dL (or 60% of serum glucose). In the instance of partially treated bacterial meningitis, the culture, and especially the Gram stain, may be nondiagnostic. The WBC count, however, should remain elevated with a predominance of polymorphonuclear leukocytes. Viral or "aseptic" meningitis seldom presents with CSF cell counts above 1,000/cu mm, and the glucose level is usually normal, although the protein value may be elevated. In a traumatic tap 400 RBCs can be "allowed" for every WBC.

In addition to the routine laboratory examinations of CSF, other tests have been described in the literature as being predictive of bacterial meningitis. These include latex fixation and counterimmunoelectrophoresis for capsular protein antigens for specific pathogens such as *H. influenzae, Neisseria meningitidis,* and *Streptococcus pneumoniae.* Serum C-reactive protein has been shown to be a sensitive and specific rapid indicator of bacterial infection. In one study, patients with bacterial meningitis had C-reactive protein levels of $17.5 +/- 2$ mg/dL whereas aseptic patients had levels ranging from 1.8 to 6.4 mg/dL. C-reactive protein using latex agglutination of CSF is also available. (C-reactive protein is not routinely used in all departments.)

CSF lactic acid of greater than 35 mg/dL is also said to be predictive of bacterial disease. Gas–liquid chromatography has also been shown to be helpful. The lactate assay, although very sensitive, has a low specificity and fails to distinguish between fungal, tuberculous, and bacterial etiologies. The chromatography method is tedious and not commonly available.

The *limulus* amebocyte lysate endotoxin assay is valuable only in identifying gram-negative infections (such as *H. influenzae*) and may be useful in determining choice of antibiotics in certain age-groups.

The most common bacterial etiology of meningitis is a function of age. From birth to 4 weeks, enteric gram-negatives (especially *E. coli*) prevail, along with group B and D streptococci. From 3 months to 3 years *H. influenzae* is the predominant organism, with the pneumococcus and meningococcus next most common. Pneumococcal meningitis and occasionally epidemic outbreaks of *N. meningitidis* are common in patients older than 3 years, although *H. influenzae* infections are becoming more common.

The timely parenteral use of appropriate antibiotics cannot be overemphasized in the therapy of bacterial meningitis. Given the variety of organisms involved and the possibility of a nondiagnostic Gram stain, initial antimicrobial therapy is usually empiric, based on the patient's age and history of exposure, if any. In the age-group from birth to 6 weeks, ampicillin, 50 mg/kg IVFD, and gentamicin, 2.5 mg/kg IVSD over 20 minutes, or IM, are given initially. In the age-group 3 months to 3 years, ampicillin (same dosage and route) and chloramphenicol (25 mg/kg IVSD) over 20 minutes are indicated. The age-group from 6 to 12 weeks of age represents a "gray area" in which pathogens are in transition. Given the frequent reports of *H. influenzae* infections in this age-group, chloramphenicol seems a more satisfactory drug than gentamicin, since enteric infections are infrequent in normal hosts after 1 month of age. Rapid serologic tests such as counterimmunoelectrophoresis or latex particle fixation can often aid in this choice. Although incidence of β-lactamase–elaborating organisms varies in different locations (20% in our institution), it is crucial to "cover" patients with chloramphenicol until the sensitivities of the organism in the CSF (not those of an organism grown from the blood) are verified. Single-drug therapy with newer-generation cephalosporins (especially cefotaxime and cefuroxime) that achieve high CSF levels and cover *H. influenzae* are undergoing clinical evaluation but are not yet accepted therapy. Some centers have used moxalactam against enteric gram-negatives, but its use in the neonate is poorly studied and its use as a single agent is contraindicated by its failure to cover group B *streptococcus*.

Prophylaxis of the patient's family with rifampin is indicated for *N. meningitidis* meningitis. Treatment of all close contacts (family members, day care center playmates) is necessary. The dosage for adults is 300 mg every 12 hours for 3 days, and for children it is 8 to 10 mg/kg every 12 hours for 3 days. The amount of IV fluids given a patient depends on the presentation. In the case discussed, routine maintenance (see Case 15) was given because the patient was slightly dehydrated (approximately 5%). Usually it is advisable to err on the "dry" side (80 to 90 mL/kg/day) to avoid exacerbation of any possible syndrome of inappropriate antidiuretic hormone that may coexist.

SUGGESTED READINGS

Clark D, Cost K: Use of serum C-reactive protein in differentiating septic from aseptic meningitis in children. *J Pediatr* 1983;102:718.

Martin WJ: Rapid and reliable techniques for the laboratory detection of bacterial meningitis. *Am J Med* 1983;119.

Twenty-month-old Male with Cough, Fever, and Seizure

CASE PRESENTATION

A 20-month-old white male was brought to the emergency department after having a generalized motor seizure at home that lasted approximately 60 seconds. There was no previous history of a seizure disorder. The child was in his normal state of good health until his mother noticed a runny nose, nonproductive cough, and a tactile temperature. Immunizations were reported as current, but none was recent. The child was on no medications. The remainder of the past medical history was noncontributory.

Vital Signs

BP: 95/50 mm Hg
HR: 150 beats/min
RR: 37/min
T: 40.6°C (105°F)
WT: 13 kg

Physical Examination

GEN: Well-developed and well-nourished alert male in no apparent distress
HEENT: *Head:* normocephalic, anterior fontanelle fibrosed. *Eyes:* PERRLA, EOM intact; normal disc and fundus. *Ears:* tympanic membranes bilaterally erythematous and dull with bulging left membrane. *Nose:* clear mucoid drainage. *Oropharynx:* minimal injection; no exudate

NECK: Supple, full range of motion; shotty posterior cervical adenopathy; negative Kernig and Brudzinski signs
CHEST: Bilateral equal expansion; clear to auscultation
CVS: Tachycardia, no murmur; pulses 2+ symmetric
ABD: Soft; nontender; normal bowel sounds; no masses
EXT: Full range of motion; no cyanosis, clubbing, or edema
NEURO: Awake and alert, irritable while examined but easily consoled by mother; deep tendon reflexes 2+ symmetric; normal sensory, motor, and cranial nerve examination
SKIN: Flushed appearance; warm and sweaty, without rash or petechiae

SUGGESTED INTERVENTIONS

1. Control fever.
   a. Antipyretic drugs:
      Acetaminophen, 10 to 15 mg/kg PO
      Drops: 60 mg/0.6 mL
      Elixir: 120 mg/5 mL
      Chewable tablet: 120 mg/1 tablet
   b. Tepid water sponging or lukewarm wet sheet for 5 to 10 minutes
2. Obtain blood specimens for CBC with differential, blood culture, C-reactive protein, glucose, electrolytes, and Dextrostix®.
3. Perform lumbar puncture.
   a. Tube No. 1 for Gram stain and culture
   b. Tube No. 2 for glucose and protein
   c. Tube No. 3 for cell count
   d. Tube No. 4: label and refrigerate
4. Perform urinalysis and urine culture and sensitivity.
5. Reevaluate patient and recheck temperature.
6. Treat otitis media.

CASE DISCUSSION

A febrile seizure is an event in infancy or childhood, usually occurring between 3 months and 5 years of age, associated with fever, but without evidence of intracranial infection or defined cause. Seizures with fever in children who have suffered a previous nonfebrile seizure are excluded. Febrile seizures are to be distinguished from epilepsy, which is characterized by recurrent nonfebrile seizures. Its prevalence ranges from 2% to 5% of young children in the United States, making it the most common convulsive disorder of early childhood.

Clinical characteristics include the following:

1. Brief, self-limited, usually generalized tonic-clonic seizure
2. Age range from 5 months to 6 years, with a peak incidence of onset at 18 to 22 months
3. Male-female ratio range: 1.1:1 to 4:1
4. Usually associated with recognizable infection (87% viral, upper respiratory tract, otitis media, roseola, shigellosis)
5. Seizure occurs during the first 24 hours of the illness and usually during the first several hours of temperature elevation.

After a convulsion with fever, the physician must distinguish if an underlying illness exists that requires immediate and specific treatment. The most urgent diagnostic decision is whether a lumbar puncture is needed to rule out meningitis. Ten to 20% of children with meningitis have convulsions with fever: these seizures are usually generalized and brief. Typical signs of meningitis (nuchal rigidity, bulging fontanelle, Kernig/Brudzinski signs, depressed sensorium) may be absent in 30% to 40% of children, especially those under 2 years of age. Some centers recommend a lumbar puncture if a child is under 2 years of age at the time of the first febrile convulsion or if the child is slow to regain baseline behavior. Even though more than 95% of lumbar punctures are normal in children with febrile seizures, if any clinical suspicion is present for meningitis, a lumbar puncture must be performed.

If the child is under 2 years of age, appears toxic, or has fever greater than 39.4°C (102.9°F), a CBC will help decide if antibiotics are indicated.

Six to 18% of children with bacteremia experience a febrile seizure. Children under 2 years of age with fever greater than 39.4°C (102.9°F) and leukocytosis of 15,000/cu mm are at a higher risk for bacteremia. Therefore, although a blood culture will not provide any immediate information, it will aid in diagnosing the cause of fever and in proposed follow-up therapy and care of the child.

Hypoglycemia is rarely associated with febrile seizures, occurring in approximately 3 in 1,000 cases. However, the glucose value is very helpful in assessing meningitis etiology. Analyzing the CSF glucose level is mandatory.

Most studies report no use for x-ray films in the evaluation of febrile seizures. Neither chest nor skull films are helpful. Computed cranial tomography has not been studied as a routine investigation in febrile seizures.

The EEG is abnormal in 90% of children on the day following a febrile convulsion. Because the EEG is expensive, rarely available in the emergency department, and of little prognostic use for recurrent febrile seizures or epilepsy, it is not indicated. The EEG can be used in the management of children with a febrile convulsion if the seizure was lengthy or focal in helping to rule out underlying structural pathology.

Asnes and associates found that only 24% of pediatricians routinely hospitalized children with a first febrile seizure if a source of fever was not found. This hospitalization allowed for close observation of the child. If the seizure was brief and nonfocal, if the child rouses to become alert and responsive, and if the examination is satisfactory except for a source of infection, hospitalization is not indicated. However, in the presence of high fever in a young infant or clinical evidence of severe illness or abnormal physical examination, hospitalization should be considered without hesitation.

Rutter and Metcalfe discovered 30% of parents who witnessed their child's febrile seizure thought the child was dying or dead. Among the 1,706 children with febrile seizures in the Collaborative Perinatal Project (NCPP) of the National Institute of Neurological and Communicative Disorders and Stroke (NINCDS), no deaths were associated with febrile seizures.

Common parental fears that need to be addressed include questions of possible epilepsy development, recurrence of the febrile seizure, and effect on intelligence. Annegens and co-workers found that 2% to 4% of children with febrile seizures later became epileptic. However, the risk of epilepsy is not uniformly distributed among children with febrile seizures. Three predictors ("risk factors") serve to identify children most likely to develop a spontaneous seizure disorder: (1) preexisting neurologic or developmental abnormality; (2) a history of seizures without fever in a member of the child's immediate family; and (3) a first febrile seizure that is focal, multiple, or lasts longer than 15 minutes. Epilepsy by the age of 7 years was found in 0.5% of children who had never had a febrile seizure, compared with 1% of those who had a febrile seizure. The incidence of epilepsy was dramatically increased to 10% in those children who had two or more "risk factors."

Overall, a third of children who have a febrile seizure experience at least one recurrence. Of those, one half had two or more and 9% had three or more recurrences. The only consistent important factor in predicting the likelihood of recurrence was early age at onset. The younger the child at first attack of febrile seizure, the more likely was the chance of recurrence. Of those recurrences, almost one half of the second attacks occur within 6 months of the first seizure, and almost three fourths occur within the first year after the initial febrile seizure.

In the NCPP, febrile seizure patients were compared with their normal siblings on IQ testing with Wechsler Intelligence Scales for Children (WISC). There was no effect on IQ or academic performance at age 7 in those children of normal ability and intellect prior to the first febrile seizure. Neither febrile seizure recurrence or length of seizure over 30 minutes was associated with any intellectual deficit.

The need for seizure prophylaxis is a controversial topic. The NIH Consensus Statement on Febrile Seizures concluded that in view of the benign nature and outcome of most febrile seizures, there was no need for medication. They further concluded that anticonvulsants *may* be considered: (1) in the presence of an abnormal neurologic examination; (2) after a prolonged (greater than 15 minutes) or focal seizure, or one associated with transient or permanent neurologic deficit; or (3) when there is a family history of nonfebrile seizures.

Perhaps the most effective prophylaxis is a full discussion with parents and care-takers of the benign nature of febrile seizures, of the management of fever, and of first aid for seizures if necessary.

SUGGESTED READINGS

Annegers JF, Hauser WA, Elveback LR, et al: The risk of epilepsy following febrile convulsions. *Neurology* 1979;29:297.

Asnes RS, Novick LF, Nealis JG, et al: The first febrile seizure: A study of current pediatric practice with implications for peer review. *J Pediatr* 1975;87:485.

Consensus Statement: Febrile seizures: Long term management of children with fever-associated seizures. *Pediatrics* 1980;62:1009.

Hertz DG, Nelson KB: The natural history of febrile seizures. *Ann Rev Med* 1983;34:453.

Joffe A, McCormick M, DeAngelis C: Why children with febrile seizures need lumbar puncture. *Am J Dis Child* 1983;137:1153.

Leviton KA, Cowan LD: Epidemiology of seizure disorders in children. *Neuroepidemiology* 1982;1:40.

Nealis JG, McFadden SW, Asnes RA, et al: Routine skull roentgenograms in the management of simple febrile seizures. *J Pediatr* 1977;90:595.

Ouellette EM: The child who convulses with fever. *Pediatr Clin North Am* 1974;21:467.

Rutter N, Metcalfe DH: Febrile convulsions—what do parents do? *Br Med J* 1978;2:1345.

Wolf SM: Laboratory evaluation of the child with a febrile convulsion. *Pediatrics* 1978;62:1074.

Case 22

Twenty-two-month-old Female with Near-Drowning

CASE PRESENTATION

A 22-month-old female who was last seen by her mother napping on the floor in the family's living room was next found 15 minutes later by a neighbor at the bottom of the family's pool, whose gate was unlocked. The child was pulled from the water without any vital signs. The actual length of submersion was unknown. The child was still warm, and the neighbor instituted CPR. Paramedics were summoned and arrived 8 minutes later instituting advanced life support. They inserted an oropharyngeal airway and started cardiac compressions and bag-mask ventilation; however, a line could not be started due to difficult venous access. They "scooped and hauled" the child Code III to the closest emergency department. Atropine, 0.28 mg, was administered sublingually during transport.

On arrival the child had an occasional idioventricular beat, was not breathing regularly, but had occasional shallow respiratory effort. The Glasgow Coma score on arrival was 3. No other history was available; the mother was so hysterical she was unable to communicate.

Vital Signs

P: 0 (occasional apical beat heard, no peripheral pulse felt)
BP: 0
RR: agonal
T: 34°C (93.2°F)
WT: 14 kg (estimated)

Case 15

Eighteen-month-old Male with Diarrhea, Dehydration, and Hypotension

CASE PRESENTATION

An 18-month-old male arrived in the emergency department with rapid pulse and tachypnea. Recent history revealed that he has had copious, continuous, foul-smelling diarrhea for the past 3 days. Although the mother states that no blood was seen in the stool, there has been significant mucus production. The child still was taking fluids orally, including full-strength cow's milk, until the prior evening; however, on this morning the child was noted to be refusing feedings and breathing more rapidly, and for the first time the mother noted slightly sunken eyeballs. Questioning revealed that the child has lost about 4 pounds from his usual 29 pounds. There has been no vomiting and no tactile or measured temperature elevation. No other family members have been ill, and there is no history of foreign travel or use of raw milk products, antibiotics, or unusual foodstuffs.

The child had been experiencing normal growth and development. All immunizations were up to date, although he was just ready for the mumps/measles/rubella immunization, which had not yet been given. There had been no prior hospitalizations; the past medical and family histories were essentially negative.

Vital Signs

T: 38.2°C (100.8°F, rectal)
HR: 170 beats/min
BP: 75 mm Hg (palpable)
RR: 35/min
WT: 11.5 kg

Physical Examination:

HEENT: *Eyes:* pupils fixed and dilated, 7 mm (post atropine); no oculospinal
reflex; Doll's eyes (deferred); fundi could not be visualized.
Oropharynx: clear

NECK: Supple; no obvious deformity; midline trachea

CHEST: Atraumatic; no respiratory effort

CVS: S_1 heard occasionally; negative S_2; no peripheral pulses

ABD: Soft; scaphoid; no mass; no bowel sounds

GU: *Pelvis:* atraumatic. *Rectum:* deferred

EXT: Appeared intact; cyanotic; cool to touch

NEURO: Flaccid; no pathologic reflexes; no clonus; no response to pain or
verbal command

SUGGESTED INTERVENTIONS

1. Place neck in sniffing position, sandbag in place.
2. Hyperventilate with bag and mask on 100% oxygen with oropharyneal airway in place.
3. Place on cardiac monitor.
4. Intubate with No. 5-0 Portex uncuffed endotracheal tube; assistant should maintain axial traction on mandibular rami and may depress the larynx (Selleck maneuver).
5. Establish large IV line, preferably 16 angiocath, peripherally; second team assigned to get large central access (subclavian, jugular, or basilic cutdown). Percutaneous femoral or saphenofemoral cutdown is permissible. Begin instillation of normal saline KVO rate. Dextrostix® first blood sample (result = 90 to 120 mg/dL).
6. Give bicarbonate, 14 mEq/L IV (most central line); epinephrine, 1.4 mL 1:10,000 IVp; atropine, 0.28 IVp; isoproterenol drip, 1 μg/kg/min to start (put 9 mg in 100 mL 5% dextrose in water, volume infusion set; start at 1 mL/hr through infusion pump).
7. Insert Foley catheter to straight drainage; obtain initial urine sample for dipstick urinalysis and culture and sensitivity; monitor output with urimeter.
8. Order lateral cervical spine x-ray (stat portable).
9. Obtain blood specimens for CBC, electrolytes, BUN, creatinine, type and hold, blood culture, ABGs, and glucose.
10. Place NG tube to straight drainage; Gastroccult® first sample.
11. Order chest x-ray.
12. Start crisis intervention with family/social services.
13. Admit to ICU.

CASE DISCUSSION

Drowning and near-drowning are common and tragic causes of death and morbidity in the pediatric population. In southern California it is the leading cause of traumatic death in the 1- to 4-year age-group.

The entire prognosis and sequelae seem to hinge intimately on the amount of cerebral anoxia sustained (i.e. the time to get good CPR started). This case represents the many problems that the arrested infant/child presents to the emergency department physician.

The paramedics will not infrequently miss lines on small infants. In Los Angeles County, we will allow the paramedics *one* try at percutaneous insertion of an IV catheter on a child 6 years of age and under. After that it is basically "scoop and haul" to the emergency department. We similarly contraindicate esophageal obturator airways (EOA) in children age 12 and under. Appropriately, the paramedics in this case instituted an oropharyngeal airway, placed the patient in the sniffing position, and then maintained ventilation with bag and mask and circulation with external cardiac massage. For active transport we favor the two-finger thrust method (although there is higher iatrogenic morbidity, it is the only method feasible when moving the patient) and the two-thumb cephalad (method of Thaler) technique for the supine patient. Neck precautions should be taken on all drowning victims when the event was unwitnessed because cervical spine injury cannot be ruled out. The paramedics are allowed to administer atropine sublingually to a patient without an IV line. This patient's bradyarrhythmia (certainly due to hypoxia) was an indication for this drug, so it was given at a dosage of 0.02 mg/kg (minimum dose is 0.15 mg), estimating the weight to be 14 kg.*

On arrival to the emergency department, the patient had agonal respirations, a very slow idioventricular rhythm, and a Glasgow Coma score of 3. The physician initiated cervical spine precautions by sandbagging the patient's neck. We believe this is a very adequate method, especially in the very young child or infant. We find that the "Philadelphia" or "California" collar is very hard to place in children in the smaller age range (under 4 years) and interferes markedly with cardiac compression and other important procedures. We generally like to start off the arrest resuscitation in small children and infants by turning them upside down and letting gravity drain the oropharynx, but this is contraindicated with suspicion of cervical spine injury. If an upper airway foreign body is suspected, we favor direct visualization with a laryngoscope and extraction with McGill forceps (pediatric) in hand. If this fails, we try the chest compression technique of ejecting the foreign body, followed by abdominal thrust (Heimlich maneuver). This latter procedure has a very high morbidity from abdominal complications but must not

---

*We estimate weight from age by doubling the age and adding 10 kg. This applies for all children over age 1 year. In children under 1 year of age we use half the age in months added to 4.0 kg.

be withheld from a child if chest compression (or direct extraction with a laryngoscope) fails.

After suctioning of the airway and adequate mask hyperventilation, a No. 5-0 uncuffed endotracheal tube was placed under direct vision with a straight blade laryngoscope. The formula to be remembered is (18 + age in years)/4. If this is forgotten, simply compare the tubes available to the child's small finger diameter or the diameter of his nares: this accurately predicts the appropriate diameter for the endotracheal tube. We use uncuffed tubes for all children under 8 years of age. Blind nasotracheal intubation is virtually impossible in this age range. The endotracheal tube position should be confirmed by auscultating both chests and stomach. Watch for adequate chest movement or, conversely, gastric distention. *Always* confirm endotracheal tube position with chest x-ray, since this gives more information than the actual physical examination. The correct length of passage from mouth to just above the carina is 20% of the crown-rump distance, but this is never measured during a "code." Always confirm with a radiograph. The tube should be suctioned well and a Luken's trap specimen taken for culture and sensitivity.

The lifeline considerations are very important, and very difficult, in the pediatric arrest. A "two team" approach should always be adopted in the critically ill or injured pediatric patient. The first team starts the first line with as large an angiocath as is possible in a peripheral vein. We find the antecubital vein ideal. Normal saline should be the first fluid hung, but kept "KVO" so that the minimum free water is transferred into the patient. This may become important if cerebral edema develops; however, occasionally in drowning (especially in salt water) the vascular volume is depleted and volume challenge is tried; in this case full-strength crystalloid is the appropriate fluid to use. As the needle goes in it is hoped that adequate blood samples can be obtained. This blood sample should be immediately subjected to the Dextrostix® test to detect treatable hypoglycemia: if so, push 1 to 2 mL/kg of 50% dextrose in water and change the IV to 5% dextrose in normal saline.

The second team starts looking for central venous access. As soon as the first line is secure, the pharmacologic treatment of this patient's idioventricular rhythm includes an empiric 1 mEq/kg push of sodium bicarbonate (2 mEq/kg may be given if the initial transport time was in excess of 15 minutes) and additional atropine and epinephrine, in an attempt to accelerate this slow ventricular focus to one of higher origin (i.e., junctional or sinoatrial). The correct dosage of atropine was given above. The dosage of epinephrine for cardiac arrest, fibrillation, vascular collapse, and severe bradyarrhythmias is 0.1 mL/kg, given as the 1:10,000 dilution IVp. If no line is in, it may be given down the endotracheal tube, in which case we take the correct amount and expand it to 5 mL saline. Finally, since our patient only partially raised her pulse (50 beats/min) to these interventions, an isoproterenol (Isuprel®) drop was started for its chronotropic and inotropic effects. The correct dosage range of isoproterenol is 0.05 to 0.5 μg/kg/min. The physician treating the child in this case study selected 0.1 μg/kg/min to start, and this is fine. Most emergency department physicians get very flustered when asked to infuse children with "μg/kg/min" dosage amounts. The "rule of sixes" presents a simple method of solving this dilemma. The "rule of sixes" states to infuse an amount of "*n*" micrograms per kilogram per minute (μg/kg/min) of drug "D," place in milligrams (mg) a quantity of drug "D" equivalent to six times the weight (kg) of the child (6 × kg) in 100 mL of fluid in a volume infusion set, and then set the infusion pump to "*n*" mL/hr. This will administer exactly the amount of *n* μg/kg/min. Correction can easily be made if the desired amount is *0.n* μg/kg/min, where now the weight is multiplied by 0.6, and added to 100 mL volume infusion set, and then the pump is set at *n* mL/hr to administer *0.n* μg/kg/min. In this case study, the infusion target was *0.1* μg/kg/min of isoproterenol where *0.n* was 0.1. Accordingly, 0.6 × 14 = 8.4 mg or 9 mg of isoproterenol was put in 100 mL of IV fluid and run at 1 mL/hr. This (*n*=1) ensures 0.1 μg/kg/min. Since the range of correct dosing of Isuppel has a ceiling of 0.5 μg/kg/min, the infusion may be incrementally increased to a maximum of 5 mL/hr. The extra beauty of the rule of six is that the fluid infused in accurate dosing of the drug is not overexcessive in terms of allowable volume (i.e., we do not drown the child while infusing the right amount of drug).

The patient in this case responded partially to this treatment, with pulse rate accelerating nicely to 95 beats/min with nice narrow complexes (i.e., supraventricular focus), but blood pressure still remained low at 65 mm Hg. A quick estimate of acceptable blood pressure in children (over 1 year of age) is 70 mm Hg + weight (kg), so we would accept 70 + 14 = 84, and therefore this child was clearly subnormal or hypotensive.

A central venous pressure (CVP) line was started, via the left subclavian approach and was of appropriate caliber, 16 F, so that a Swan-Ganz catheter could be inserted later in the ICU. As a general rule we never start pulmonary arterial wedge pressure monitoring in the emergency department. It is too time consuming and should be appropriately done in the ICU.

We favor the subclavian approach here, because we have a large experience in its placement; the technique is different from the adult placement, but it is beyond the scope of this case study to go into detail. We have a very low rate of complication to this procedure. Other sites for CVP access are via a percutaneous femoral line, a saphenofemoral cutdown, a right external jugular stick (frequently enters the central system in children), and finally an internal jugular site. The initial CVP will be helpful in deciding if this persistent hypotension is on a hypovolemic basis (low CVP) or a cardiogenic-pulmonary basis (high CVP).

Initial CVP on our patient was high at 15 mm Hg, so next a dolbutamine drip was started at 5 μg/kg/min (see rule of six). The range for this drug is 1 to 20 μg/kg/min, and it is favored over dopamine for its pulmonary vasodilating capability.

ABGs after intubation were pH, 7.20; Po_2, 45 mm Hg; and Pco_2, 30 mm Hg. The patient was hooked to a volume ventilator, with FIo_2 initially set at 100%, total volume at 150 mL (10 mL/kg); RR at 30/min, and PEEP at 10 cm. The next ABGs returned were pH, 7.32; Po_2, 75mm Hg; and Pco_2, 35 mm Hg. The pressure was now at 85 mm Hg (systolic, Doppler). PEEP was upped to 17 cm.

The chest x-ray showed infiltration of the right lower lobe, the endotracheal tube in good position right above the carina, and the tip of the left subclavian catheter in the right atrium–superior vena caval junction. No pneumothorax was seen, and there were no gross abnormalities. The lateral cervical spine was completely normal down to the C7 level, so sandbags were removed and an NG tube was placed; Gastroccult® was negative, and the tube was hooked to low continuous suction.

A urine sample was obtained and was hematest − ; the subsequent flow rate was 25 mL/hr, well above the 1 mL/kg/hr minimum (oliguric) parameter. Macroscopic and microscopic examination proved negative.

All hematologic and metabolic values came back normal, and the child was switched to 5% dextrose in 0.2 normal saline, and run at two-thirds calculated maintenance volume, as a prophylaxis to cerebral edema. (See Case 15 for calculating maintenance volumes.)

The child left for the PICU with normal blood pressure and on a ventilator.

SUGGESTED READINGS

Drowning and Near-Drowning. In Shoemaker W (ed): *Critical Care Manual*, sec.I(F)10. Los Angeles, Society of Critical Care Medicine, 1983.

Modell et al: Clinical course of 91 consecutive near drowning victims. *Chest* 1976;70:231.

Peterson B: Morbidity of childhood near drowning. *Pediatrics* 1977;59:364.

Case 23

Three-year-old Female with Large Burn, Stridor, and Wheezing

CASE PRESENTATION

A 3-year-old female was extricated from a burning apartment wherein she sustained burns to a large area of her trunk, buttocks, legs, and perineum. There was considerable smoke in the room, and the child presented in marked respiratory distress with stridor and wheezing. She was awake and very agitated.

Past medical history revealed a long history of bronchial asthma, with her last visit to the emergency department 1 week prior, at which time she was restarted on theophylline, given as a slow release preparation, at a dosage of 20 mg/kg/day. She was also on 30 mg/day of prednisone. Her immunizations were up to date, and there were no known drug allergies. One parent was killed in the fire, and the other was not injured. There were no other siblings. The child was rushed to the emergency department in the arms of a bystander rescuer, who was first on the scene. He noted a fetid odor of burning plastics in the room that was burning. There were no apparent prior injuries or burns in this child. No other history was immediately available.

Vital Signs

BP: 85 mm Hg (palpable)
P: 155 beats/min
RR: 45/min
T: NA
WT: 16 kg (estimated)

Physical Examination

HEENT: *Head:* singed nasal and facial hair; singed brows. *Eyes:* PERRLA; EOM intact; fundi normal; marked conjunctivitis. *Ears:* tympanic membranes clear. *Nose and Throat:* soot in the nares and oropharynx.

NECK: Supple; marked inspiratory stridor over larynx; midline trachea

CHEST: Inspiratory and expiratory wheezing; prolonged expiratory phase with I:E = 3:7; bilateral symmetrical sounds; no rales; no rubs; + + subcostal retraction; intracostal retraction; nasal flaring; no pulsus paradoxicus

CVS: Tachycardia; no murmur; no gallop rhythm; no rub; loud S_1

ABD: Soft; absent bowel sounds; no mass; no rebound, nontender; no costovertebral angle tenderness; no palpable liver, kidneys, or spleen

GU: *Rectum:* heme$^-$; normal tone

EXT: No cyanosis, clubbing, or edema

NEURO: Awake, in great distress; + + + pain; not cooperating for status examination; responds appropriately to all stimuli; normoreflexive

SKIN: Partial-thickness burns to face, excluding nape, and left cheek; entire neck involved, not completely circumferential; anterior chest with partial-thickness burns; posterior chest spared; anterior abdomen involved some with full-thickness burns on lower left abdomen (approximately 2%); perineum involved with partial-thickness burns on left anterior thigh and both buttocks. Anterior aspects of both arms affected with partial-thickness burns. No burns circumferential; both axillae spared; positive corneal involvement of left eye. Initial total estimated burn = 51% (includes 2% full thickness).

SUGGESTED INTERVENTIONS

1. Administer oxygen, 5 L/min, via nasal prongs.
2. Place on cardiac and Doppler monitors.
3. Insert two large-bore IVs to left antecubital area and left hand veins. Dextrostix® blood sample (result = 90 to 120 mg/dL).
4. Intubate with orotracheal tube (No. 5-0 Portex tube, uncuffed); premedicate with atropine, 0.32 mg IVp.
5. Begin infusion with Ringer's lactate. Initiate at 205 mL/hr (103 mL/hr/line).
6. Suction orotracheal tube with Luken's trap for culture and sensitivity.
7. Place Foley catheter (or infant feeding tube). Perform urinalysis and urine culture and sensitivity; hook to urimeter for continuous output monitoring.

8. Place NG tube: aspirate; Gastroccult®; hook to continuous low suction.
9. Apply sterile, cool saline dressings to all burns.
10. Obtain blood specimens for ABGs, CBC, theophylline level, electrolytes, BUN, glucose, and creatinine.
11. Administer meperidine (Demerol®), 16 mg IV.
12. Administer aminophylline (bolus as per theophylline level), and begin immediate 16 mg/kg/hr continuous infusion.
13. Administer methylprednisolone sodium succinate (Solu-Medrol®), 32 mg IVp.
14. Administer aqueous penicillin G, 800,000 units IVSD, volume infusion set.
15. Order portable upright chest x-ray.
16. Stain corneas with fluorescein.
17. Admit or arrange transport to burn center.

CASE DISCUSSION

Trauma is the leading cause of death in the pediatric population. Burns cause a significant proportion of that mortality.

This 3-year-old child presented with a large significant burn as well as respiratory complications, including laryngeal burn/edema and exacerbation of her underlying asthma by smoke inhalation.

The immediate life-saving interventions included oxygenation on arrival, initiation of fluid resuscitation, and then controlled rapid intubation for impending airway obstruction from laryngeal edema secondary to airway burn.

Large IV lines were instituted immediately, and nonburned sites were selected. In cases in which all potential IV sites are burned, it is much more important to get the volume infusing, then to avoid possible infection by cannulation through a burned area. These sites are sterile initially, but it is true that they colonize with bacteria at a higher rate subsequent to admission. Delay must be avoided at all costs in establishing good large-bore IV infusions.

The airway was secured with a No. 5-0 uncuffed Portex endotracheal tube. We use the formula:

$$(\text{Age} + 18)/4 = \text{Endotracheal tube size (mm)}$$

So for this 3-year-old child:

$$(3 + 18)/4 \cong 5 \text{ mm}$$

However, for those who are not facile with formulae and equations, pick a tube that approximates the size of the child's little finger or the diameter of his or her nares.

In general, we favor tubes without cuffs for children 8 years of age and under; this is to prevent complications of tracheal stenosis, tracheal perforation, and postextubation obstructive airway syndromes. As always, in a child with a pulse rate less than 200 beats/min, we favor premedication with atropine, 0.02 mg/kg, to prevent the strong vagal deceleration associated with the procedure of intubation. If the calculated amount (0.02 × kg) is less than 0.15 mg total atropine, then this "minimum amount" is administered. It is well reported that low-dose paradox exists with atropine. It is parasympathomimetic in low dosages instead of parasympatholytic. This child received 0.02 × 16 = 0.32 mg.

The child was ventilating adequately on her own, so the tube was hooked to 100% T-tube blow-by pending ABG determinations.

The strategy of intubating early in the course of airway burn is very wise. Waiting for manifest obstructions commits the physician to a crash tracheostomy, which is a very morbid procedure in the pediatric population. The added morbidity and mortality from this procedure, as well as greater susceptibility to septicemia with a tracheostomy (especially one done emergently) make this intervention highly undesirable. The moment stridor is detected is the moment the intubation should be planned!

Fluid resuscitation is the next most important life-saving priority, since with the magnitude of this burn, loss of integument will lead to a major loss of body fluids. In general, a burn (excluding superficial partial-thickness "first-degree" area) in excess of 15% total surface area indicates fluid replacement in childhood. This parameter is adjusted down to 10% or greater in the infant 1 year of age or less. Any pediatric patient with a full-thickness burn in excess of 5% should be fluid resuscitated.

As in all trauma patients, Ringer's lactate is the number one selection for infusion. There is no change in this policy for the seriously burned child. As always, with initial cannulation, a drop of blood should be checked with Dextrostix® to detect hypoglycemia or hyperglycemia. For hypoglycemia, push 1 to 2 mL/kg of 50% dextrose in water and start with 5% dextrose in Ringer's lactate. We concur that colloid should not be used in the first 24 hours of therapy.

Initial hypotension (not usually seen within the first hour in the seriously burned patient) should be treated either by opening the Ringer's lactate wide (severe hypotension) or by the bolus technique (20 mL/kg boluses) for borderline hypotension.

The burn area calculation follows standard "rule of nines" with some modification for age. The adult rule gives 9% to the head, 36% to the trunk (4 × 9%), 9% to each upper extremity, and 18% (2 × 9%) to each leg. This adds up to 99%, and 1% more is added for the perineum.

The pediatric correction can be simplified as follows. In the infant and small child the head has more surface area relative to the rest of the body and basically is "borrowed" from the surface of the legs. So the percentage added to the head is generally subtracted from the legs. A rule of thumb states that the bonus added to the head and therefore subtracted from the legs follows the following formula:

Bonus % = 10/A, where A is the age in whole integers at the child's next birthday

For this 3-year-old, the "bonus" percentage = 10/3 ≅ 3. Therefore, the maximum surface area of the head is 9 + 3 = 12%, and 1.5 points are subtracted from each leg. The surface area of a 3-year-old's leg is 18 − 1.5 = 16.5%.

From this formula it probably is not worth correcting the basic rule of nines formula for any child over 3 years of age. For any infant under age 1 year, A = 1.

Many burn formulas exist for the calculation of initial rate of infusion of volume. We favor the Baxter formula:

24-hour resuscitation volume (mL) = (2 mL/kg/% burn area)
+ daily maintenance volume

or the Parkland formula:

24-hour volume = 4 mL/kg/% burned area,

whichever gives the most fluid volume per 24 hours!

The limitation of the Parkland formula for small children is that for burns less than 50%, the calculated amount is actually less than the daily maintenance volume. So it is wisest to calculate using both formulas and then choose the one that provides the most volume. Since this patient was 51%, the calculations would be close:

Baxter: (2 × 16 × 51) = 1632 mL + maintenance volume = 24-hour volume requirement
= 1632 + [1000 + 50(16-10)] (see Case 18)
= 1632 + 1300
= 2932 − mL/24 hr

Parkland: 4 × 16 × 51 = 3264 mL/24 hr

Therefore, choose the Parkland amount. As with most repletion formulas for children the first half is given in the first 8 hours. Therefore, the total hourly infusion rate for the two lines established was:

3,264/(2 × 8) = 204 mL/hr, or 102 mL/hr each line

(*Note*: all volume given in first 24 hours is full-strength crystalloid—either normal saline or Ringer's lactate—for both maintenance and burn surface area.)

It must be emphasized that these are guidelines for initiation of fluid resuscitation. Parameters of perfusion such as blood pressure, pulse rate, urine output, level of consciousness, and skin perfusion must all be evaluated to determine the efficacy of these suggested flow rates. There should be no hesitation to advance volume rates for falling perfusion or signs of decreasing intravascular volume.

An infant feeding tube (No. 5 F) was used for a urinary catheter. We find these safer in infants and smaller children, whereas Foley catheters are harder to pass and tend to cause strictures. The initial urine sample was sent for urinalysis and for culture and sensitivity. The catheter was hooked to a urimeter for continuous monitoring. We accept nothing less than 2 mL/kg/hr as adequate urine output for the burned pediatric patient. Any reduction should indicate inadequate volume status and should encourage volume bolus and increased hourly infusion rates. Acute tubular necrosis and myoglobinuric failure are commonly seen in large burns. The treatment of acute tubular necrosis is the same as volume depletion; however, myoglobinuric failure dictates alkaline forced diuresis. The suspicion of myoglobinuria or hemoglobinuria is raised by a macroscopic urinalysis positive for "blood" in excess of the observed RBCs on the high-power microscopic field. The diagnosis is confirmed by agar gel diffusion of the urine (this will differentiate hemoglobinuria from myoglobinuria). Also, in myoglobinuria there is an elevated serum creatinine and aldolase level and a reversed BUN/creatinine ratio. This child was negative for pigment in her urine (dipstick).

An NG tube is absolutely essential. Pediatric burn victims hyperventilate secondary to their hypovolemia (and in this case from respiratory disease) and develop gastric dilatation very rapidly. In addition, reduced splanchnic blood flow causes an early ileus. These factors both predispose to vomiting and aspiration. The early amelioration of stress ulceration (Curling's ulcers) includes NG suction, observation for "coffee grounds" or actual blood aspirant, and administration of hourly antacids per NG tube.

Cool, sterile compresses were applied to all burns. We favor no topical antibiotic dressing (e.g., Silvadene®, Silver Nitrate®, Xeroform®, Sulfamylon®) be placed until the initial resuscitation has been completed and the surgeons have evaluated the patients themselves.

This patient had no circumferential full-thickness burns of the chest, extremities, or neck. Any suspicion of neurovascular compromise in the extremities or respiratory restriction from the chest necessitates immediate consultation with the surgeon to consider escharotomy to release tension. No anesthetic is necessary for these procedures since they are, by definition, full thickness and, therefore, painless. Large hemorrhage, however, can be precipitated by these incisions, especially in small children, so maintain adequate volume infusion and make sure adequate blood has been cross-matched and is ready for use on demand.

Blood was drawn and sent off for initial type and cross-match; CBC with platelet count; ABGs, with carboxyhemoglobin level and cyanide determination; serum electrolytes; BUN; creatinine; glucose; and theophylline level.

Hemolysis is seen frequently in patients with large burns. The need for actual transfusion must be balanced against the high hematocrit of hemoconcentration secondary to fluid loss. So, as in this entire discussion, adequate volume (Ringer's lactate) resuscitation is critical. The type and cross-match anticipates any future transfusion. Obviously, because hepatitis and acquired immune deficiency syndrome must be considered, transfusions are to be reserved for absolute indications. The initial CBC will document baseline values, with specific regard to hematocrit and platelet counts. Hemoconcentration and hemolysis will alter these values. Disseminated intravascular coagulation, seen frequently in burns, might be picked up early by a decrease in the platelet count.

ABG determination was crucial in this patient with underlying asthma, now complicated by smoke inhalation and upper respiratory stridor. ABGs are very useful in any seriously burned patient, since the presence of a small metabolic acidosis must be considered hypovolemia until proven otherwise and would mandate an acceleration of volume infusion. Serial ABG determinations can nicely monitor, along with other parameters mentioned above, the success of the volume resuscitation. In this patient, however, the ABGs took on extra significance because of the exacerbation of her asthma. A normal or elevated Pco_2 would certainly be indicative of impending respiratory failure. She was intubated early for the stridor, but respiratory failure secondary to severe bronchospasm could have been a separate independent indication. Her initial ABGs were pH, 7.50; Po_2, 240 mm Hg; and Pco_2, 28 mm Hg. Thus, ventilation and oxygenation were adequate.

The patient was burned in a closed space, as well as in a room described as acrid with smoke from burning plastics. Carboxyhemoglobin levels and cyanide levels were ordered to rule out these complications. The 100% oxygen and intubation were initial treatments, but considerations of hyperbaric oxygenation (for carbon monoxide poisoning) and sodium nitrite infusion (for cyanide toxicity) must be entertained. This patient's carboxyhemoglobin level was benign (3%), and there was no detectable cyanide. Some centers now recommend initiating sodium nitrite infusion for any victim of closed space burn until the cyanide is returned for analysis.

The serum theophylline level was wisely obtained early because of the need, obvious on presentation, for IV theophylline therapy. Our policy on patients already on theophylline is to initiate the continuous infusion of Aminophylline® (1 mg/kg/hr) immediately but to wait for the measured serum theophylline level to adjust the blood level to a therapeutic level. If the child has not been on previous theophylline preparations in the past 24 hours, we would bolus the full 6 mg/kg (Aminophylline®); however, if the child has not abstained for at least this period of time, we wait for the measured level. We then calculate the bolus on the following correction: each 1 mg/kg bolus will raise the serum level 2 μg/mL.

This patient's level came back 8 μg/mL. Since we aim for a therapeutic level of 15 μg/mL, the appropriate bolus for her was (15 − 8)/2 = 3.5 mg/kg. Accordingly, shortly after her continuous infusion of 16 mg/hr (1 mg/kg/hr) was started, it was augmented with a 56-mg bolus (3.5 mg/kg × 16 kg) infused over 10 minutes.

This patient had been on corticosteroids, and it is well reported that when such patients are stressed (her serious burn *and* bronchospasm from smoke inhalation) they have very poor intrinsic steroidal response. Accordingly, she was given a pharmacologic dose, parenterally, of methylprednisolone sodium succinate (Solu-Medrol®). We favor 2 mg/kg IVp. Incidentally, we use this dosage in any patient admitted with status asthmaticus. An alternate glucocorticoid is dexamethasone, 0.5 mg/kg, IV, given initially and then repeated every 6 hours.

Pain control is a significant part of the management, unless, of course, the patient has sustained complete full-thickness burns—a very dismal situation usually. We use meperidine (Demerol®), 1 mg/kg, IV. Untoward reactions such as respiratory depression (this patient was already intubated) or hypotension can be reversed with naloxone (dose equal to 0.01 mg/kg—minimum, 1 ampule).

As prophylaxis for streptococcal burn sepsis, an initial infusion of aqueous penicillin G, using 50,000 units/kg, was administered. The use of penicillin prophylactically is still controversial.

This child's tetanus immunizations were up to date, so no prophylaxis was indicated. Burns are high risk for tetanus contamination, so any child without a full prior immunizing series of three shots is given a tetanus toxoid. Similarly, any child who has not had his last booster within the past 5 years should receive one. Any patient with two or less prior boosters is given a tetanus immune globulin (TIG) shot, unless the burn is fresh (under 24 hours old) *and* he has had two prior boosters. (A full adult dose of 250 units IM for all pediatric patients, administered intramuscularly is frequently favored.)

By this point the patient was resuscitated with her airway secure and large bore IVs in place and infusing; nasogastric suction and urinary drainage were effected; and medications were administered to treat the bronchospasm and to provide prophylaxis against infection and adrenal suppression.

A chest x-ray was obtained to check tube placements and cardiorespiratory status.

For completion, the corneas were stained with fluorescein to rule out corneal burns/ulcers. Positive reactions should dictate an immediate ophthalmologic consultation.

This patient was admitted by the surgery service to the pediatric ICU. Any patient with a burn of this magnitude seen in a community emergency department should be transported (with physician in attendance) to a regional burn center or pediatric critical care center.

SUGGESTED READINGS

Crowley RA, Dunham CM (eds): Burns. In *Shock Trauma/Critical Care Manual*. Baltimore, University Park Press, 1982.

Goldfarb W, Pruitt A: Burns. In Shoemaker WC, Thompson WL (eds): *Critical Care State of the Art*. Fullerton, CA, Society of Critical Care, 1980.

Pruitt BA: The burn patient: Initial care and management. *Curr Probl Surg* April 1979;16:162.

Two-year-old Female Who Swallowed Hearing Aid Battery

CASE PRESENTATION

A 2-year-old female was witnessed by her parents to swallow a hearing aid battery prior to emergency department presentation. The battery belonged to her father. She initially coughed and since the ingestion has vomited all liquids and solids offered. There is no drooling or respiratory distress. She does not appear to be in pain. There is no history of surgery or stricture of the esophagus. The mother was in the room at the time of the ingestion. There is no previous history of an ingestion, broken bone, or burn.

Vital Signs

HR: 130 beats/min
RR: 30/min
BP: 95/60 mm Hg
T: 37°C (98.6°F)
WT: 14 kg

Physical Examination

HEENT: *Head:* NCAT. *Eyes:* conjunctiva clear; PERRLA; EOM intact. *Ears:* clear tympanic membranes. *Nose:* clear nares. *Oropharynx:* clear with no drooling
NECK: Supple
CHEST: Lungs clear to percussion and auscultation; no retractions or stridor
CVS: Regular rate and rhythm without S_3, S_4, or murmur; full pulses

ABD: Soft; normal bowel sounds; no masses, tenderness, or hepato-
              splenomegaly
EXT: No bony or joint abnormalities
NEURO: Grossly normal
SKIN: No cyanosis or lesions

SUGGESTED INTERVENTIONS

1. Keep patient NPO.
2. Keep the patient upright.
3. Order x-rays to include an anteroposterior and lateral neck view, chest film, and kidney/ureter/bladder.
4. Request ENT consultation.

CASE DISCUSSION

Between the ages of 1 and 4 years swallowing of foreign bodies is very common. Coins are the most common objects ingested. In recent years an increasing number of small disk-shaped alkaline batteries have been ingested. This parallels their increasing use in radios, watches, hearing aids, cameras, and calculators. In general, if the coin is located below the diaphragm there is a 90% to 95% chance it will pass through the GI tract without complication in 7 to 10 days. The most common sites for objects to impact are in areas of natural narrowings, such as the cricopharyngeus, thoracic inlet, aortic arch, lower gastroesophageal sphincter, pylorus, ligament of Treitz, and ileocecal valve. The fear exists that any impaction of a smooth object can lead to ulceration, erosion, and perforation, resulting in mediastinitis, peritonitis, abscess formation, and fistulas. Coins are relatively inert substances so that current recommendations are for immediate intervention only if the coin is located above the diaphragm or the patient is symptomatic. The management of disk alkali battery ingestions has become more controversial since they contain toxic substances. Their main ingredients include alkali such as potassium hydroxide and/or heavy metals such as mercury or cadmium.

Several mechanisms exist for the toxicity of the disk-shaped batteries. As in any foreign body ingestion, impaction may cause pressure necrosis and perforation. The alkali used is usually in a high concentration, 20% to 45%. This alkali may be released not only by actual rupture of the battery but also by leakage across a damaged seal. Once in contact with mucosa the alkali causes liquefaction necrosis and possible perforation of the viscus. The potential risk is greater if the battery is lodged at a single site rather than free floating and therefore diluted. In addition, impaction allows even a slow leak to have a more cumulative effect. Another mechanism of injury is tissue electrolysis. When the battery is in a conducting media such as in the GI tract there may be a current generated external to the battery causing electrical injury to the mucosa. Heavy metals such as mercury also have a potential for toxicity if systemically absorbed. Finally, there is the potential for mechanical intestinal obstruction.

Acutely, the symptoms of ingestion of a battery are similar to the symptoms of any other form of ingestion. The child may refuse to take food and complain of pain or discomfort on swallowing. The child may be drooling and vomiting with or without blood. An esophageal foreign body may impinge on the trachea so that respiratory distress may be prominent on presentation and mimic a foreign body aspiration. Patients with an ingestion that has been missed acutely may present with chronic pain, vomiting, and infections such as peritonitis, mediastinitis, or abscess formation.

The initial approach to ingestion of a disk-shaped battery is similar to that for ingestions of other foreign bodies. If there is respiratory distress, oxygen should be applied and the airway secured. The patient should be suctioned as needed and kept NPO. The patient should be encouraged to sit upright to prevent aspiration and impingement on the trachea and to assist the force of gravity. Ipecac ingestion and gastric lavage are contraindicated not only because of the alkali but also because of the risk of airway obstruction at the time of regurgitation of the foreign body. Neck, chest, and abdominal x-rays should be obtained. Anteroposterior and lateral neck films will help distinguish the location in the trachea versus the esophagus. A flat object like a coin will usually lie in the frontal plane if it is in the esophagus and in the sagittal plane if it is in the larynx. Determination of heavy metal levels should be performed if the battery has opened or been in place longer than a day to determine if chelation therapy is necessary.

A study of 56 ingestions of disk-shaped batteries showed that impaction in the esophagus was the uniform predictor of severe morbidity. It is uniformly agreed in the literature that once a battery is lodged in the esophagus it should be removed immediately. The method of removal is a matter of choice. The earlier the removal, the fewer are the sequelae. All patients should be followed up in 2 to 3 weeks after removal of the esophageal battery to evaluate for possible stricture formation.

There is considerable controversy about the management of a battery ingestion once it has passed out of the esophagus. The majority of the available data support a very benign course for battery ingestions beyond the esophagus. Although any symptomatic patient should be handled aggressively, the majority of cases only require supportive measures and observations as an outpatient, with spontaneous passage occurring within 7 to 10 days without complication. Even for batteries that have spontaneously opened in the lower GI tract, surgery is rarely indicated, with enema removal being the treatment of choice. If the battery is below the level of the diaphragm the patient should be observed for development of symptoms and the stool searched for the battery. If after 3 days the battery has not been passed, another x-ray should be taken. If the battery has progressed from its initial site, the patient and stools should again be observed. If the battery has not progressed, then a surgical consultation should be obtained since the risk of perforation may increase the longer the duration of impaction at a given site. The patient should be reevaluated immediately if symptoms of obstruction, erosion, or perforation should develop. Cathartics may help to decrease the transit time.

The National Electrical Manufacturers Association has published a master cross-referenced index of all ingestible batteries made by the three major manufacturers. If the serial number of the battery is known, then the contents can be determined. All ingestions require an evaluation of the family situation since the incidents of poisonings and ingestions are directly correlated with the degree of stress within a family.

This patient was found on x-ray to have a battery lodged in the distal third of the esophagus. An ENT consultation was obtained, and the battery was removed by esophagoscopy on the day of presentation. She was discharged the following day. She had no evidence of stricture formation at her 3-week follow-up.

SUGGESTED READINGS

Giordano A, Adams G, Boies L, et al: Current management of esophageal foreign bodies. *Arch Otolaryngol* 1981;107:249.

Litovitz T: Button battery ingestions. *JAMA* 1983;249:2495.

Mofenson H, Greensher J, Caraccio TR, et al: Ingestion of small flat disc batteries. *Ann Emerg Med* 1983;12:88.

Rumack, B, Rumack C: Disk battery ingestion. *JAMA* 1983;249:2509.

Temple D, McNeese M: Hazards of battery ingestion. *Pediatrics* 1983;71:1090.

Volteler TP, Nash JC, Rutledge JC: The hazard of ingested alkaline disk batteries in children. *JAMA* 1983;249:2504.

Case 25

Twenty-six-month-old Male with Fever, Cough, and Tachypnea

CASE PRESENTATION

A 26-month-old black male presented to the emergency department with a 3-day history of repeated nonproductive cough, temperature spikes to 39.4°C (103°F), and marked increase in respiratory rate. There was a questionable family history of sickle cell trait. The child was previously well, had had no major illnesses, and was the product of a normal full-term pregnancy and noncomplicated spontaneous vaginal delivery. He had no perinatal complications, went home on the second day, was breast-feeding, and had no respiratory disease, jaundice, or perinatal fevers. All immunizations were current. He had had no allergies or no atopic dermatitis or asthma.

On further questioning the mother stated that the child was becoming slightly more irritable, was beginning to refuse feedings, but was still on solid foods supplemented with milk. There was no vomiting nor diarrhea and no weight loss, and the child was urinating normally. The mother did note intermittent shaking chills.

Vital Signs

T: 39°C (102.2°F)
P: 135 beats/min
RR: 45/min
BP: 85 mm Hg (palpable)
WT: 16 kg

Physical Examination

HEENT: *Eyes:* PERRLA; EOM intact; conjunctivae pale, without inflammation; fundi flat; no retinopathy. *Ears:* right tympanic membrane red
and slightly bulging; left tympanic membrane normal; canals normal.
Oropharynx: well hydrated without exanthem

NECK: Supple; multiple anterior cervical lymph nodes; negative Kernig and
Brudzinski signs; no strider; midline trachea

CHEST: Rapid respiration; good tidal effort; crepitant rales; right posterior
lung fields; subcostal retractions; no nasal flaring

CVS: Increased P_2; normal S_1; no murmur, gallop rhythm, or rub; normal
point of maximal impulse

ABD: Soft; decreased bowel sounds; no mass; no palpable liver, kidneys,
or spleen; no rebound; no costovertebral angle tenderness

EXT: Slight acrocyanosis; no clubbing; no edema; pale nail beds

NEURO: Alert, oriented x3, normal motor, sensory, cerebellar, and cranial
nerve evaluation; normoreflexive

SKIN: Normal turgor; no exanthem

SUGGESTED INTERVENTIONS

1. Administer oxygen, 3 L/min via nasal prongs.
2. Start IV with 5% dextrose in 0.2 normal saline at 80 mL/hr (1.5 times
   maintenance).
3. Place on cardiac monitor.
4. Obtain blood specimens for CBC, C-reactive protein, blood culture, electrolytes, glucose, sickle preparation, and hemoglobin electrophoresis.
5. Order ABGs.
6. Order chest x-ray.
7. Perform urinalysis.
8. Consider admission.

CASE DISCUSSION

This febrile, tachypneic, coughing black child with auscultated rales certainly
suggests the diagnosis of bacterial pneumonia. The differential diagnosis may
include sinusitis, asthma, tuberculosis, aspirated foreign body, tracheoesophageal
fistula, gastroesophageal fistula, lung abscess, congenital or acquired heart disease, bronchiectasis, pulmonary infarct, or tumor. The acute nature of the disease,
absence of wheezing, nasal drainage, history of aspiration, chronic weight loss,

fatigue, inanition, hemoptysis, and prior murmur make the majority of these unlikely.

We find that the examination of the chest in young infants may be misleading in that frequently children under 3 years of age may have a paucity of auscultatory findings, when in fact the chest x-ray shows definite infiltration. Also, the converse occurs with atelectasis (from various causes) mimicking pneumonic infiltration (rales); however, the x-ray is clear or perhaps has some streaking in the perihilar/peribronchiolar distribution.

The finding of pulmonary infiltration in a child with sickle hemoglobinopathy (SS, SC, SO, SJ) is extremely important, always dictates admission, and frequently indicates exchange transfusion. The differentiation of pulmonary infarction from pneumonic infiltration by standard laboratory and radiographic methods may prove difficult. Pulmonary infarction, though, is rarely seen in sickle cell patients under 5 years of age.

The patient in this case study was started on oxygen immediately because he was in moderate respiratory distress; he also had a cardiac monitor placed, which is wise since it may be the first tipoff to significant hypoxia.

The IV was run at one and one-half times maintenance to guarantee good hydration. Laboratory studies were obtained to address the issue of hemoglobinopathy, hematologic status, and underlying metabolic condition. The blood culture is frequently positive in the febrile child and may give the first and only clue to the underlying pathogen involved. Study of sputum specimens is invariably unrewarding. We routinely obtain blood cultures on all children 2 years of age and under who present with a temperature of 39°C (102.2°F) and above.

A WBC count over 15,000/cu mm and a positive C-reactive protein are prime indicators of bacterial disease. The CBC can give a first indication of the chronicity of hypoxia (elevated hematocrit) or demonstrate underlying anemia (low hematocrit), such as shown in sickle cell anemia.

The ABGs, on 3 L, came back pH, 7.56; Po_2, 70 mm Hg; and Pco_2, 28 mm Hg. The sickle preparation was negative, the WBC count was 19,500/cu mm, and the hemoglobin/hematocrit was 12 g/dL/36%. Differential blood count showed 65 segments, 20 bands, 8 lymphocytes, 3 monocytes, 2 basophils, and 2 eosinophils; toxic granulations were seen. The mean corpuscular volume was normal, and the platelet count was 200,000/cu mm. The C-reactive protein value was elevated. All other metabolic studies were negative.

Routine urinalysis showed 10 to 15 WBCs and was otherwise negative. The urine specimen was sent for culture and sensitivity.

The chest x-ray, obtained in the radiology department with the patient transported with a nurse and still on oxygen, showed infiltration of the right middle lobe and right lower lobe. There was no pleural effusion; no pneumatoceles were seen, and there was no pneumothorax. Apices were clear, and heart size and configuration were all normal. No perihilar calcifications nor nodes were discernible.

The diagnosis was probable pneumococcal pneumonia. The negative Sickle-dex® and absence of significant anemia (in a fairly well hydrated patient) make the diagnosis of sickle hemoglobinopathy unlikely. Electrophoresis was nevertheless sent off.

The etiologic consideration of pneumonias in this age-group (3 months to 5 years), in a nonimmunocompromised patient, place viral disease highest on the list. The leading culprits would be respiratory syncytial virus and parainfluenza, and in epidemic bouts, adenovirus and influenza A/B. The high fever, high WBC counts, elevated C-reactive protein, and lobar infiltration make viral pneumonia unlikely, however, in this patient.

Tuberculosis is always a possibility. The child had no history of exposure or of tine or Mantoux testing. A test with purified protein derivative of tuberculosis was placed in the emergency department.

Mycoplasm infection would be highly unlikely in a child under 5 years of age or in a nonimmunocompromised host. The positive C-reactive protein is atypical of most *Mycoplasma* pneumonias, as is the high WBC count.

Of the leading agents, bacteria must be considered the etiology in this case until proven otherwise. Pneumococci is the most likely if the disease is truly bacterial, with *Hemophilus* a good second choice. The finding of a "hot" tympanic membrane makes *Hemophilus* more likely. The dissemination and gravity of pneumococcal infections in actual sickle cell patients must not be forgotten. Most sicklers now receive Pneumovax® at age 2 years.

Streptococci pyogenes pneumonia is unlikely to develop de novo and is usually associated with a much more toxic course. It has a very painful pleuritic component, as well as early development of pleural effusion, which is usually very large in volume.

Staphylococcal pneumonia is very unlikely to develop in a previously well, nonhospitalized, nonimmunosuppressed patient.

With pneumococci and *Hemophilus* the leading considerations for bacteria etiology, the emergency department physician in this case elected to give the patient one shot of procaine penicillin, 600,000 units IM, and started him on cefuroxime, 200 mg/kg/day IVSD, with a loading dose of 50 mg/kg.

As stated above, the physician also placed a Mantoux TB skin test, ordered chest physical therapy, and admitted the patient to the infectious disease ward, with respiratory isolation.

SUGGESTED READINGS

Gisburg CM, Howard JB, Nelson JD: 65 cases of *Hemophilus* pneumonia influenza b. *Pediatrics* 1979;64:283.

Long SS: Treatment of acute pneumonia in infants and children. *Pediatr Clin North Am* 1983;30:297.

Murphy TF, Hendersen FW: Pneumonia: An 11 year study in pediatric practice. *Am J Epidemiol* 1981;113:12.

Thirty-month-old Male with Fever and Limp

CASE PRESENTATION

A 2½-year-old black male presented to the emergency department with a 2-day history of fever to 38.9°C (102°F) and pulling at his ears. Approximately 8 hours previously, his mother noted that he was not moving his right leg well and refused to walk or stand. There is no history of trauma, previous joint swelling, rashes, or antecedent infectious symptoms. There have been no recent immunizations or injections. The child has never been tested for sickle cell disease.

Vital Signs

BP: 90/65 mm Hg
HR: 120 beats/min
RR: 30/min
T: 38.7°C (101.7°F)
WT: 15 kg

Physical Examination

GEN: Well-developed, well-nourished, irritable child who on examination was lying with his right leg flexed at the hip, abducted, and externally rotated
HEENT: *Eyes:* PERRLA; EOM intact. *Ears:* red tympanic membranes, bulging with poor mobility and landmarks in mastoid area without erythema or swelling
NECK: Supple; moderate shotty cervical adenopathy

CHEST: Clear to auscultation
CVS: Pulses +2 bilaterally; heart tones normal; no rub or gallop rhythm
ABD: Soft; nontender; no hepatosplenomegaly, masses, or costovertebral angle tenderness
GU: Normal appearance; no swelling or lesions
EXT: Normal upper extremities and spine without point tenderness; right hip diffusely tender with mild swelling of the proximal thigh, increased warmth, and mild erythema over the inguinal region without lymphadenopathy, masses, or point tenderness; marked increased tenderness with movement of the hip joint; no point tenderness of remainder of pelvis or lower extremity; no obvious trauma or bruising atrophy of the muscles
NEURO: Awake; alert; normal motor and sensory examination; cranial nerves and deep tendon reflexes within normal limits

SUGGESTED INTERVENTIONS

1. Obtain blood specimens for CBC, ESR, blood culture and sensitivity, sickle prep, and glucose evaluations.
2. Order anteroposterior and frog-leg views of the pelvis and right lower extremity.
3. Request orthopedic consultation.
4. Prepare patient for a diagnostic hip joint aspiration with fluid sent for WBC count and differential, Gram stain, culture and sensitivity, and glucose test.

CASE DISCUSSION

In diseases of the hip, early diagnosis and appropriate therapy is essential to prevent further problems with the hip joint after the initial insult has been treated. Increased pressure in the hip joint from accumulated fluid can lead to destruction of the femoral epiphysis, acetabulum, or vessels, with subsequent chronic hip problems.

This is a classic presentation for a septic arthritis in a febrile child with swelling of the thigh and pain on motion of the limb. Positioning with flexion, abduction, and external rotation at the hip alleviates some of the pressure in the joint space, which is small compared with the knee. The WBC count and ESR are usually elevated, and in the majority of cases there is an evident source for the infection (e.g., skin wounds, otitis media, pneumonia). This child's ESR was 95 mm/hour; his WBC was 15,000/cu mm with shift to left.

Septic arthritis must be differentiated from a variety of other conditions associated with fever, including a superficial cellulitis or adenitis, osteomyelitis, toxic synovitis, juvenile rheumatoid arthritis, retroperitoneal abscess, discitis, and sickle cell crisis. Hip aspiration differentiates a septic hip from these other conditions. In neonates, pseudoparalysis may be the first clue to a septic arthritis. A septic hip may be confused with femoral venous thrombosis, but again the aspirated joint fluid will aid the diagnosis, since x-ray films are difficult to interpret due to the lack of ossification of the epiphysis. They may not differentiate among septic hip, toxic synovitis, and early juvenile rheumatoid arthritis, in which local soft tissue and capsular swelling are seen. A frequent, notable finding in a septic joint is lateral-superior displacement of the proximal femur or, in neonates, displacement of the medial femoral metaphysis from the acetabulum. A careful look at the bones for lucencies heralding possible osteomyelitis is indicated, although this radiologic finding occurs 10 to 14 days into the course of that infection. Untreated osteomyelitis can lead to a septic arthritis.

All children with septic arthritis *must* be admitted for IV antibiotic therapy and arthrotomy.

Organisms responsible for septic arthritis can be spread by direct invasion, as in the case of osteomyelitis extending into the joint, or hematogenously, as is the case seen most often with *Hemophilus influenzae,* commonly in children from 1 to 18 months of age. *Staphylococcus* and gram-negative rods are common in newborns, with *Streptococcus, H. influenzae,* gonococcus, and *Salmonella* also found in older children. It is important to screen black children for sickle cell anemia, since this disease predisposes them to *Salmonella* infection. Direct trauma from puncture wounds, including femoral venipuncture, must be considered in the search for a point of entry. Tuberculosis is a possible pathogen in septic arthritis, although usually the presentation is less acute. IV antibiotic therapy should be combined with arthrotomy to decompress the joint. Antibiotics alone are not sufficient for treatment of a septic joint. Some experts advocate arthrotomy within 6 hours of aspiration of pus from a joint to minimize the possibility of permanent damage.

Antibiotic choice prior to culture results should be dictated by Gram stain of aspirated joint fluid. When no bacteria are seen, treatment should be based on the age of the patient. In the neonatal period gram-negative enterics and gram-positive cocci are the usual pathogens, so combined treatment with methicillin and gentamicin would be indicated. Older infants and children frequently have *H. influenzae* or staphylococcal infections and therefore should be treated initially with methicillin and chloramphenicol. Treatment should be changed to the safest effective drug once bacteriologic test results are known. Septic arthritis of the hip should be treated intravenously for 4 weeks.

This child had a negative sickle prep and was not anemic. His hip aspiration appeared purulent, and Gram stain revealed pleomorphic gram-negative rods. The Quellung reaction was positive for *H. influenzae.* He was started on ampicillin and chloramphenicol, pending results of sensitivity studies, and was scheduled for hip arthrotomy.

SUGGESTED READINGS

Nelson JD: The bacterial etiology and antibiotic management of septic arthritis in infants and children. *Pediatrics* September 1972;50:437–440.

Nelson WE: *Textbook of Pediatrics,* ed 11. Philadelphia, WB Saunders, 1979, pp 716–717, 776.

Schaller JG: Arthritis and infections of bone and joints. *Pediatr Clin North Am* 1977;24:775–790.

Two-and-one-half-year-old Male with Vomiting and Lethargy

CASE PRESENTATION

A 2½-year-old male presented to the emergency department with a 1-day history of lethargy and vomiting. He was well until 3 days ago when he developed a runny nose and fever. He was taken to his pediatrician who diagnosed an upper respiratory tract infection and recommended aspirin for fever control. He was improving until the previous night when he began vomiting and becoming more lethargic. The mother also reported decreased fluid intake and urine output. The emesis was nonbilious and not associated with abdominal pain. He had a normal bowel movement the morning of presentation. Besides lethargy he appeared at times to be hallucinating. There is no history of head trauma, neck pain, drug ingestion, or seizures. The mother denied giving any medications except aspirin. She has been giving one adult aspirin every 6 hours for the past 3 days. The past medical history and review of systems were noncontributory. Immunizations are up to date. There is no previous history of ingestions, accidents, or broken bones.

Vital Signs

HR: 160 beats/min
RR: 40/min
BP: 95/60 mm Hg
T: 38°C (100.4°F)
WT: 14 kg
M²: 0.6

Physical Examination

GEN: Slightly lethargic and dehydrated male

HEENT: *Head:* NCAT. *Eyes:* sunken; clear conjunctiva; PERRLA; EOM intact; flat discs with normal venous pulsations. *Ears:* normal tympanic membranes. *Oropharynx:* injected with dry mucous membranes

NECK: Supple without adenopathy; negative Kernig and Brudzinski signs

CHEST: Rapid, deep respirations with no retractions, rales, or wheezes

CVS: Tachycardia without S_3, S_4, or murmur; full pulses

ABD: Normoactive bowel sounds; no tenderness, masses, or hepatosplenomegaly

GU: *Rectum:* soft stool in the ampulla, heme negative. *Genitalia:* normal male

EXT: No bony or joint abnormalities

NEURO: Slightly lethargic but arousable to verbal stimuli and will answer questions; cranial nerves intact; gag reflex intact; reflexes bilaterally symmetric with downgoing toes; normal motor, sensory, and coordination examinations

SKIN: No acute lesions with normal skin turgor

SUGGESTED INTERVENTIONS

1. Administer oxygen, 5 L/min.
2. Place on cardiac monitor with rhythm strip.
3. Measure heart rate and blood pressure in the supine and sitting positions.
4. Begin cooling measures.
5. Obtain blood specimens for CBC, platelet count, electrolytes, BUN, creatinine, glucose, ABGs, SGOT, SGPT, ammonia, prothrombin time, blood culture, salicylate level, toxicology screen, and Dextrostix® (result = 100 mg/dL).
6. Establish an IV line. Hang 5% dextrose in normal saline to start.
7. Administer naloxone (Narcan®), 0.01 mg/kg/min, 1 ampule, IVp.
8. Give 50% dextrose at a dose of 1 g/kg IV if the glucose value is less than 60 mg/dL.
9. Place NG tube for gastric lavage with normal saline, keeping the head down and turned to the left. Save aspirant for toxicologic screen.
10. Administer activated charcoal, 30 g per NG tube after lavage is completed.
11. If there are postural changes (a decrease in systolic blood pressure greater than 20 mm Hg or an increase in heart rate greater than 20 beats/min going from supine to sitting), give normal saline, 20 mL/kg, as a bolus. If there are no changes, begin IV with 5% dextrose in normal saline; run at 1½ maintenance until full laboratory values are available. Therefore begin infusion at 75 mL/hour (see discussion below).

12. Obtain urine sample for urinalysis and toxicologic screen.
13. Order chest x-ray.
14. Perform lumbar puncture with opening pressure.
15. Start alkalinization with sodium bicarbonate at a dose of 0.5 to 1.0 mEq/kg/hr and titrate to a urine pH of greater than 7.5 (see discussion below).
16. Call for a pediatric consultation and arrange for admission to a pediatric ICU for close observation and laboratory evaluation.

CASE DISCUSSION

Salicylate ingestions remain an important problem for the emergency department physician. The trend has been away from acute aspirin ingestions and toward chronic and therapeutic overdoses. The decrease in acute ingestions is partly due to the packaging laws that place limits in the number of chewable tablets per bottle and require child-resistant caps. Chronic or therapeutic overdoses account for about half of hospitalizations but 80% of deaths due to aspirin ingestions. Chronic overdoses occur in several ways. The parents, as in this case, may give an adult aspirin rather than a children's aspirin or give it too frequently. Many cold remedies contain aspirin, which the parents may not be aware of. Furthermore, the diagnosis of chronic salicylism may be delayed because of symptoms and signs resembling those for which the aspirin is being given. It is important to ask specifically about aspirin since many parents do not consider it a medication.

Aspirin is usually absorbed quickly. However, when taken in large doses it may inhibit gastric emptying and form concretions, which may delay absorption up to 24 hours. It is usually fully distributed within 6 hours. It is primarily metabolized by the liver, with some renal excretion of salicylic acid. The kinetics of elimination are important because the major pathways are saturable. As a result, with increasing dose, the time required to eliminate a given fraction of a dose increases and the blood levels increase more than proportionately. In addition, the renal excretion of salicylic acid becomes more important. This renal clearance is sensitive to changes in pH. At a higher pH, the salicylic acid becomes ionized and trapped in the renal tubule.

Salicylic acid causes many physiologic derangements. It causes a direct stimulation of the CNS respiratory center, resulting in tachypnea and respiratory alkalosis. This stimulation is independent of the oxygen or carbon dioxide content of the blood. The decrease in carbon dioxide causes an increase in renal bicarbonate excretion, resulting in a diminished buffering capacity. This primary respiratory alkalosis is predominately seen in adolescents and adults but may also be seen in younger children with mild to moderate ingestions.

A metabolic acidosis is more frequently seen in younger children. Salicylates uncouple oxidative phosphorylation, inhibit the Krebs cycle, inhibit aminotransferases, and increase fat mobilization and ketone production. As a result of these metabolic derangements there is an elevation of lactic acids, organic acids, and ketones leading to a high anion-gap acidosis. The severity of the acidosis increases with decreasing age and increasing dose in an acute ingestion and with increasing severity of the chronic administration. Clinically, this may result in Kussmaul respirations, vomiting, decreased peripheral perfusion, cardiac dysfunction, disseminated intravascular coagulation, and altered mental status.

Hypoglycemia may also be seen as a result of increased metabolic demands and decreased glucose production. This is more common in the younger child. The CNS is particularly susceptible to hypoglycemia. CSF glucose levels may be depressed even with a normal peripheral glucose level. As a result of hypoglycemia the child may appear agitated, lethargic, or comatose with seizures, tachycardia, pallor, and diaphoresis. Because of the decrease in adenosine triphosphate production, energy is released in the form of heat, leading to hyperpyrexia.

Another important sequelae of salicylate intoxication is water and electrolyte losses. The increase in metabolism and heat production causes increased cutaneous insensible losses. The organic aciduria secondary to the inhibition of aminotransferases causes obligate water and solute losses. Pulmonary insensible losses are increased as a result of the elevated respiratory rate. This dehydration is exacerbated by vomiting and decreased intake. The dehydration may be severe with losses up to 4 to 6 L/M^2 in severe salicylate toxicity. Clinically, the dehydrated patient may present with lethargy, tachycardia, decreased peripheral perfusion, hypotension, sunken eyes, dry mucous membranes, decreased skin turgor, and oliguria. Hypokalemia is often present secondary to vomiting and renal losses. A normal serum potassium value in the presence of acidosis usually represents a total body potassium depletion. As a result the child may have an ileus, emesis, and arrhythmias. Hyponatremia or hypernatremia may be present.

Salicylate intoxication also causes a diffuse capillary fragility and capillary leak. This, plus the alterations in energy metabolism, contribute to the development of cerebral and pulmonary edema. Other sequelae are ammonia and liver enzymes and altered hemostasis with an elevated bleeding time and prothrombin time, although frank bleeding is rare.

The initial signs and symptoms, the estimated dose of ingestion, and the measurement of the salicylate level all serve to assess the severity of an acute aspirin ingestion. However, in cases of chronic salicylism the clinical picture is the most useful guideline. As discussed above, the signs and symptoms are nonspecific and may mimic the signs and symptoms of the illness for which the aspirin is being given so a high index of suspicion is necessary. The differential diagnosis is extensive. With alterations in mental status, an antecedent viral infection, vomiting, hepatomegaly, elevated ammonia levels, and cerebral edema, salicylism may closely resemble Reye's syndrome. A history of fever and mental status changes is also suggestive of meningitis. Pneumonia may be suggested by an increased respiratory rate and fever. With a predominance of GI symptoms and signs the diagnosis may be confused with an acute gastroenteritis, bowel obstruction, or hepatitis. Metabolic disorders such as ketotic hypoglycemia and other drug ingestions such as alcohol must also be considered.

The estimated amount of drug ingested may be predictive of the severity of the clinical syndrome in acute ingestions. Ingestions of less than 150 mg/kg are usually benign and asymptomatic. Ingestions in the range of 150 to 300 mg/kg cause mild to moderate toxicity with hyperpnea, lethargy, hypoglycemia, and acidosis. Ingestions greater than 300 mg/kg usually show more severe symptomatology, and ingestions greater than 500 mg/kg may be lethal. Such guidelines do not apply to chronic poisonings, but toxicity may result when doses greater than 100 mg/kg/day are ingested for more than 2 days.

To assess most accurately the severity of an acute salicylate intoxication, a salicylate level 6 hours post ingestions is best. The level can then be correlated with severity and prognosis by using the Done nomogram. Levels taken before 6 hours cannot be used to predict severity. The level cannot be used in chronic salicylism since a level less than 30 mg/dL may be associated with severe symptoms. Concretions may be formed when large numbers of capsules or tablets are ingested, resulting in the absorption of aspirin over several hours. As a result, serial salicylate levels may be necessary before a patient is discharged from the emergency department. Other indicated blood tests include ABGs, CBC, platelet count, electrolytes, BUN, creatinine, glucose, prothrombin time, SGOT, ammonia, toxicologic screen, and blood culture.

A urine sample for an analysis and toxicologic screen should also be obtained. If there is no evidence of an acute rise in intracranial pressure but the patient is lethargic and/or febrile, a lumbar puncture is indicated. Depending on the neurologic findings a CT scan may be needed. A chest x-ray should be obtained if pneumonia or pulmonary edema is suspected. A Phenistix® with a change in color to purple indicates a level greater than 70 mg/dL. A positive ferric chloride test just indicates the presence of salicylates.

The principal causes of morbidity and mortality are cerebral edema and cerebral depression, pulmonary edema, and cardiac dysfunction. A cardiac monitor to check for arrhythmias and any evidence of hypokalemia, as well as supine and sitting blood pressures and heart rates, should be done. If there is an intact gag and the patient is awake, ipecac should be given. If the gag is compromised or the patient is lethargic, gastric lavage with normal saline should be done using the largest possible NG tube while maintaining adequate airway protection. Both should be followed by activated charcoal. Many schema exist for fluids, calling for an initial hydration rate of 10 to 15 mL/kg for 1 to 2 hours then 4 to 8 mL/kg/hr until the salicylate level normalizes. Since pulmonary edema and cerebral edema, as well as dehydration, are important parts of the pathophysiology of salicylate intoxication, both overhydration and underhydration should be avoided. The percent of dehydration based on clinical parameters should be established. If there are orthostatic changes, an initial bolus of normal saline, 20 mL/kg, should be given. If there are no orthostatic changes, as in this patient, fluids should be started at maintenance plus replacement. The following "scorecard" describes the correct calculation of fluid and electrolyte orders.

"Scorecard" (see Case 15) developed for this 14-kg child, with 10% dehydration acquired over 3 days; serum electrolyte values returned with sodium = 140, potassium = 3.8, chloride = 95, and bicarbonate = 13.

	Water	*Sodium*	*Potassium*
Maintenance:	$1,000 + (4 \times 50) = 1,200$ mL	$3 \times 14 = 42$ mEq	$2 \times 14 = 28$ mEq
Replacement:	$10\% \times 14,000$ mL $= 1,400$ mL		
	Extracellular (60%) $= 840$	$0.84 \times 135 = 114$ mEq	
	Intracellular (40%) $= \underline{560}$		$0.56 \times 160 \times \frac{1}{2}$
	1,400 mL		$= 45$ mEq
Totals	2,600 mL	156 mEq	73 mEq
(per liter)	(1,000 mL)	(60 mEq)	(28 mEq)

Fluid orders, therefore, should indicate to start with 5% dextrose in 0.4 normal saline and run initially at 162 mL/hour. Each liter of fluid should contain 28 mEq of potassium chloride, as long as the patient is not anuric. The flow rate is based on the principle of administering the first half of the day's allotment in the first 8 hours (see Case 18). Of course, these values must be corrected for any boluses of fluid given in the emergency department. If alkalinization is included (see below), sodium administered as sodium bicarbonate should be debited from the scorecard, as appropriate.

If the patient is hypoglycemic, 50% dextrose should be given at 1 g/kg IV bolus. Ten or 5% dextrose should be started, depending on the patient. The serum glucose value also needs to be monitored closely. Hyponatremia or hypernatremia may be present. Therapy with vitamin K may be indicated if the prothrombin time is prolonged or if there is frank bleeding.

Alkalinization is indicated to promote trapping in the renal tubule of the ionized form. Start with 0.5 to 1.0 mEq/kg/hr, watching serum pH and potassium levels carefully. The goal is to achieve a urine pH greater than 7.5. This is difficult to achieve in children, especially with the aminoaciduria. The sodium content needs to be considered when deciding on IV fluids.

Dialysis is indicated only if renal failure is present, if there are persistent CNS symptoms and acidosis, or if there is persistent deterioration. Because of the severe fluid and electrolyte disorders and cerebral edema, admission to a pediatric ICU is indicated.

This patient had an initial salicylate level of 35 mg/dL and pH of 7.27. A bicarbonate drip was maintained for 18 hours, and there was improvement in hydration and mental status over the next 48 hours. The serum potassium level fell to 2.5 mEq/L during treatment and the patient required additional potassium. He was transferred to the floor after 36 hours and was discharged after 4 days with no sequelae.

SUGGESTED READINGS

Done A: Aspirin overdosage: Incidence, diagnosis and management. *Pediatrics* 1978;62(suppl):890.

Levy G: Clinical pharmacokinetics of aspirin. *Pediatrics* 1978;62(suppl):867.

Temple A: Acute and chronic effects of aspirin toxicity and their treatment. *Arch Intern Med* 1981;141:364.

Temple A: Pathophysiology of aspirin overdosage toxicity with implications for management. *Pediatrics* 1978;62(suppl):873.

Winchester J: Extracorporeal treatment of salicylate or acetaminophen—Is there a role? *Arch Intern Med* 1981;141:370.

Case 28

Three-year-old Male with Fever, Stridor, and Drooling

CASE PRESENTATION

A 3-year-old male presented in the emergency department with a 1-day history of fever and noisy breathing. The patient was well until the morning of admission when he developed a fever. He also complained of a sore throat and did not want to eat. About 6 hours after the onset of the fever he was noted to be drooling and making noise on inspiration. The parents deny any lethargy, cough, or runny nose. He has no history of foreign body ingestion or aspiration. There is no previous history of intubation or stridor. His immunizations, including DPTs, are up to date.

Vital Signs

HR: 160 beats/min
RR: 40/min
T: 40°C (104°F)
BP: 90/60 mm Hg
WT: 16 kg

Physical Examination

GEN: Alert, but stridorous, toxic, and anxious child who prefers to sit with his jaw thrust forward
HEENT: Drooling; further examination deferred
NECK: Midline trachea; stridor (inspiratory) heard over trachea

155

CHEST: Suprasternal and subcostal retractions; breath sounds good bilaterally with no rales or rhonchi; prominent transmitted upper airway noises

CVS: Regular rate and rhythm with no S_3, S_4, or murmur; full peripheral pulses

ABD: Deferred

EXT: Deferred

NEURO: Alert; further examination deferred

SKIN: Good perfusion with no cyanosis

SUGGESTED INTERVENTIONS

1. Keep child upright and preferably with the mother at all times. Using a mask held close to but not over the child's mouth, waft oxygen past the nares. Have a physician skilled in airway management present with the child at all times.
2. Notify anesthesiology, otolaryngology, and critical care personnel immediately.
3. Place equipment for bag and mask ventilation, intubation, and tracheostomy at the bedside. Endotracheal tubes of appropriate size, as well as 0.5 mm and 1.0 mm smaller than estimated by the patient's age should be available. Endotracheal tube size can be estimated by the following formula: (age in years + 18)/4. For this patient (3 + 18)/4 is approximately 5.0 so endotracheal tubes sizes 4.0, 4.5, and 5.0 should be available.
4. Keep the patient NPO.
5. Administer a trial of 0.25% racemic epinephrine, nebulized.
6. Keep manipulation and examination of the patient to a minimum. Do not attempt venipuncture.
7. Obtain a lateral neck x-ray. The lateral neck film should be obtained in the emergency department with a physician in attendance and the child in a sitting position.
8. Transport the patient to the operating room with a nurse and physician in attendance and with equipment for intubation.
9. Once the child is in the operating room establish an IV line and secure the airway by intubation or tracheostomy.
10. Obtain cultures of the blood and epiglottis and administer antibiotics. Appropriate choices include the combination of ampicillin at a dosage of 800 mg (200 mg/kg/day divided every 6 hours) and chloramphenicol at a dosage of 400 mg (100 mg/kg/day divided every 6 hours) or cefuroxime alone at a dosage of 400 mg (75 mg/kg/day divided every 8 hours). The antibiotics are administered intravenously.

CASE DISCUSSION

Epiglottitis is the second most common infectious etiology of stridor and accounts for 1 of every 1,000 pediatric admissions. It is a life-threatening disease for which early diagnosis and prompt institution of treatment are essential to ensure survival.

Epiglottitis has been described in all ages from infancy to adulthood, but the majority of cases occur in ages 3 to 7 years. It can occur year round, but it is most common in the winter. *Hemophilus influenzae* type B is the most important pathogen accounting for 80% to 90% of cases. Group A β-hemolytic *Streptococcus* and *S. pneumoniae* have also been implicated as etiologic agents.

Involvement of the epiglottis results from bacteremic spread of *H. influenzae.* Inflammatory edema begins on the lingual surface of the epiglottis and rapidly spreads to the aryepiglottic folds, the arytenoids, and the entire supraglottic area. As a result, the caliber of the airway is markedly decreased. There are two proposed mechanisms for the acute airway obstruction seen in patients with epiglottitis. Some authors propose that the loose swollen epiglottis may be sucked into the glottis while others believe that pooled secretions accumulate and plug the already compromised airway.

The onset is usually abrupt with the duration of illness rarely exceeding 24 hours and possibly being as short as 6 hours prior to presentation. Usually fever is the first symptom noted and frequently is as high as 40°C (104°F). Shortly after onset of the fever the patient may complain of a sore throat (50% of cases) and have decreased oral intake. The voice may seem muffled, although hoarseness is rare. Stridor is present in virtually all patients secondary to the narrowed airway. Drooling may develop as the edema interferes with swallowing. Coughing is very rare.

On physical examination the child appears toxic. His mental status may range from agitated to stuporous, depending on the degree of hypoxia and sepsis. The child may prefer a sitting position with his jaw thrust forward to maximize the airway patency. The temperature is usually elevated. Tachycardia and tachypnea are common. Cyanosis, retractions, and nasal flaring may be present, depending on the severity of the airway obstruction. In the child with impending total airway obstruction stridor may be absent. Cyanosis, lethargy, and marked retractions are all signs of impending respiratory arrest. Drooling is observed in 60% to 70% of patients. Twenty-five percent of patients have an associated cervical adenitis, and another 25% have pneumonia. Meningitis, pericarditis, cellulitis, and septic arthritis have all been very rarely associated with epiglottitis.

Most authors recommend that no attempt be made to examine the oropharynx and that manipulation of the patient be kept to an absolute minimum. Most hospitals have protocols for the management of patients with suspected epiglottitis. A physician skilled at airway management should be with the patient at all times. Anesthesiologic, otolaryngologic, and critical care personnel should be notified immediately. The equipment for bag and mask ventilation, intubation, and tracheostomy or cricothyroidotomy should be placed at the bedside. Endotracheal tubes one size smaller than estimated by the patient's age should be available. Endotracheal tube size can be estimated by the formula: (age in years + 18)/4. An IV line and blood work should not be attempted until the child is in the operating room, unless the child is grossly septic on presentation, a situation that immediately demands antibiotic therapy and volume resuscitation, as well as airway management. The patient should be kept NPO. A trial of 0.25% aerosolized racemic epinephrine should be tried. An occasional case of severe croup mimics epiglottitis and should reverse well with racemic epinephrine. We have seen this phenomenon occur. Racemic epinephrine does *no* harm if the underlying pathology is indeed epiglottitis. Children whose conditions clear with racemic epinephrine must be admitted. Rebound is predictable after racemic epinephrine in severe croup.

A lateral neck film should be obtained. Findings on the lateral neck film can be both sensitive and specific for epiglottitis. The film should be obtained in the emergency department with a physician in attendance and the patient in a sitting position. The radiographic findings of epiglottitis include thickening of the epiglottic tissue and aryepiglottic folds with obliteration of the vallecula and pyriform sinuses. The rounded thickening of the abnormal epiglottis gives it the appearance of an adult thumb on the anteroposterior projection. A normal epiglottis will have the configuration of an adult little finger in the lateral projection.

The x-ray has proven very useful to us in either confirming the diagnosis or indicating other processes in the differential such as foreign body, retropharyngeal abscess, bacterial tracheitis, and so on.

Because of the limits placed on the physical examination, the history is very important in the differential diagnosis of the febrile patient with stridor. Croup (laryngotracheitis) is the most common infectious cause of stridor. Sixty percent of cases of croup are caused by a parainfluenza virus. It starts as an infection of the pharynx that spreads downward to the larynx, causing edema and mucous production of the vocal cords and subglottic region. It is most common in ages 6 months to 3 years. It can be distinguished from epiglottitis in part based on clinical course. In contrast to epiglottitis, croup begins insidiously, with fever and coryza preceding the onset of stridor by 1 to 3 days. A barking cough is almost always present when the stridor begins. In epiglottitis coughing is very rare. The patient with croup is usually only mildly to moderately toxic. Drooling is usually absent, and hoarseness is frequent.

Fever, tachycardia, and tachypnea may be present in patients with either croup or epiglottitis. In addition, patients with croup may present with impending respiratory failure secondary to obstruction. The lateral neck of patients with croup is usually normal or may show dilation of the hypopharynx and/or subglottic narrowing. The epiglottis, however, appears normal.

Bacterial tracheitis presents with a course similar to croup except that the child appears more toxic and has very purulent tracheal secretions. It is an unusual infection but most commonly occurs in younger children. *Staphylococcus aureus* is the usual causative agent. It can be distinguished from epiglottitis by the more insidious onset, often being superimposed on a preceding viral illness. The lateral neck film may show dilation of the hypopharynx and subglottic narrowing, but the epiglottis will be normal.

A child with a retropharyngeal abscess may also present with a course similar to epiglottitis. The usual pathogens are group A β-hemolytic *streptococcus,* anaerobes, and *S. aureus*. These again are uncommon infections, but most reports have been in young children. The child with a retropharyngeal abscess is febrile and toxic appearing, with stridor and drooling secondary to the abscess impinging on the esophagus and trachea. Again the clinical course may help differentiate epiglottitis from a retropharyngeal abscess. With the latter, the course is usually less abrupt with symptoms developing over several days. A lateral neck film again will be most helpful. In a patient with a retropharyngeal abscess the epiglottis will be normal and there will be increased width of the soft tissues anterior to the cervical vertebrae. In general, in a film with the neck properly extended, the width of the prevertebral soft tissues is less than one half of the width of the adjacent vertebral body.

Diphtheria, although much rarer than in the preimmunization era, is still present in sporadic outbreaks. These patients may present with stridor, drooling, and toxicity out of proportion to the fever. A careful immunization history and history of recent contacts is important. What serves to differentiate diphtheria from epiglottitis besides the presence of a grayish membrane is the less abrupt onset and presence of cutaneous lesions, myocarditis, and neurologic involvement.

Tonsillitis with or without a peritonsillar abscess very rarely presents with marked respiratory compromise. The usual pathogens are group A β-hemolytic streptococci and a muffled voice. Again the clinical course is usually insidious with 2 to 4 days of sore throat and fever. The lateral neck will show tonsillar enlargement and possible adenoidal hypertrophy, but the epiglottis will be normal.

There are many noninfectious etiologies of stridor that may be present coincidentally in the child who is febrile or be exacerbated by a viral upper respiratory tract infection. Again the history is very important in establishing whether the stridor preceded the onset of the acute febrile illness and whether the episodes of stridor have been recurrent. These noninfectious etiologies include laryngomalacia, vocal cord paralysis, tracheal web, subglottic stenosis (congenital or acquired secondary to intubation), laryngeal hemangioma or papilloma, vascular ring, and so on. Also the possibility of trauma and foreign body aspiration or ingestion always should be considered.

Treatment to maintain an adequate airway should precede any diagnostic evaluation. There are reports in which patients with epiglottitis have been successfully bagged on an emergent basis. Most authors believe that in the event of an impending respiratory arrest prior to reaching the operating room intubation should be attempted followed by emergency tracheostomy (if surgical expertise is available) or by needle cricotomy/cricothyroidotomy if a surgeon is not in attendance. The child should be escorted to the operating room by a physician and nurse with the equipment necessary to maintain the airway on an emergent basis.

Once the child is in the operating room an IV line can be placed and the larynx examined. The airway will be secured by intubation or tracheostomy. Most pediatric centers are now advocating intubation over tracheostomy. Children treated with intubation in general have a shorter hospital stay and overall less morbidity than those treated with a tracheostomy. However, the choice of intubation is predicated on having an ICU environment that can ensure 1:1 nursing and the presence 24 hours a day of an individual capable of reintubating the child if he is accidentally extubated. Careful and adequate sedation of the patient is important once the airway is secure by intubation.

In the operating room, blood cultures, CBC, and cultures from the epiglottis should be obtained. Blood cultures have been reported as positive in 65% to 90% of patients for *H. influenzae* type B. Typically the WBC count is elevated to 15,000 to 25,000/cu mm with a left shift.

The choice of antibiotics may vary depending on the hospital. Approximately 25% of *H. influenzae* are reported as resistant to ampicillin at most centers. Until recently the antibiotics of choice were a combination of ampicillin at a dosage of 200 mg/kg/day in divided doses every 6 hours and chloramphenicol at a dosage of 100 mg/kg/day in divided doses every 6 hours. Both antibiotics were continued until culture and sensitivity data were known. More recently, cefuroxime has been used for serious *H. influenzae* infections alone at a dosage of 75 mg/kg/day in divided doses every 8 hours.

This child was kept in the emergency department for a lateral neck film, which showed a swollen epiglottis. He was escorted to the operating room without problems. He was nasotracheally intubated and started on ampicillin and chloramphenicol. His blood culture grew *H. influenzae* sensitive to ampicillin and the chloramphenicol was discontinued. He was afebrile after 24 hours and extubated at 48 hours. He was discharged on oral antibiotics 4 days after admission with sequelae.

SUGGESTED READINGS

Bottenfield G, et al: Diagnosis and management of acute epiglottitis: Report of 90 consecutive cases. *Laryngoscope* 1980;90:822.

Diaz J, Lockhart JC: Early diagnosis and airway management of acute epiglottitis in children. *South Med J* 1982;75:399.

Faden H: Treatment of *Haemophilus influenzae* type b epiglottitis. *Pediatrics* 1979;66:402.

Fulginiti V: Infections associated with upper airway obstructive findings. *Pediatr Infect Dis* 1983;2:533.

Lewis J, Gartner J, Galvis A: A protocol for management of acute epiglottitis. *Clin Pediatr* 1978;17:494.

Podgone J, Bass J: The "thumb sign" and the "little finger sign" in acute epiglottitis. *J Pediatr* 1978;88:154.

Wetmore R, Handler S: Epiglottitis: Evolution in management during the last decade. *Ann Otol* 1979;88:822.

Three-and-one-half-year-old Male with Abdominal Pain and Hematemesis

---

CASE PRESENTATION

A 3½-year-old male, weighing 17 kg, ingested a bottle of 35 ferrous sulfate capsules, each containing 50 mg of elemental iron. The child ingested the material approximately 1 hour prior to admission to the emergency department. He was unsupervised at the time, and the mother was out shopping. The child has received no prior immunizations and has had one admission for aspirin ingestion 1 year prior. He has severe abdominal pain on admission and had one episode of scant vomitus, which was "coffee ground" in appearance.

Vital Signs

BP: 90/55 mm Hg
HR: 110 beats/min
RR: 42/min
T: 37°C (98.6° F)
WT: 17 kg

Physical Examination

HEENT: *Eyes:* PERRLA; EOM intact; normal fundi, sclerae, and corneas. *Ears:* normal tympanic membranes. *Throat:* without enanthem; no burns; well hydrated. Gag reflex intact
NECK: Supple; full range of motion; no nodes; midline trachea; no stridor; negative Kernig and Brudzinski signs
CHEST: Clear to bases; no wheezes, rhonchi, rales, or rub

CVS: Normal rhythm; no gallop rhythm, rub, or murmur; normal S_1 and S_2

ABD: Diffusely tender; absent bowel sounds; no mass; no involuntary guarding; no costovertebral angle tenderness; no liver, kidney, or spleen palpable

GU: Soft, well-formed stool; heme $++$; normal tone; nontender

NEURO: Awake; alert; normal motor, sensory, cranial nerve, cerebellar, and reflex evaluation

SUGGESTED INTERVENTIONS

1. Administer ipecac, 15 mL + 200 mL of water. Save emesis for Gastroccult® and toxicology study.
2. Establish IV line with normal saline, KVO.
3. Place on cardiac monitor.
4. Obtain blood specimens for toxicologic screen, CBC, ABGs, Dextrostix® (result = 90 to 120 mg/dL), serum iron and TIBC, glucose, electrolytes, BUN, liver function tests, and type and hold.
5. Order urinalysis.
6. Order portable abdominal x-ray.
7. Order toxicologic screen of urine and emesis.
8. Give deferoxamine (Desferal®), 680 mg, IM (40 mg/kg). Observe urine for next 2 hours.
9. Admit patient for continued observation and decision to continue Desferal® therapy.
10. Notify child abuse team.

CASE DISCUSSION

The child ingested a toxic dose of elemental iron (i.e., in excess of 80 mg/kg). Note ferrous sulfate contains 20% elemental iron, so each 250-mg capsule contains 50 mg. This patient therefore ingested $(35 \times 50)/17$ kg = 102 mg/kg of elemental iron.

It has further been noted that onset of abdominal symptoms (abdominal pain, bloody emesis, and/or diarrhea) within 6 hours of ingestion has almost 100% sensitivity to toxic blood levels (i.e., in excess of 300 mg/dL); of course, discomfort of ipecac-induced emesis must be differentiated from these symptoms, but ipecac rarely has prolonged emesis, and almost never with pain, and *never* with bloody stool or hematemesis. The abdominal distress of this youngster must be considered consistent with toxic iron levels.

Because he had no contraindications to induced emesis (i.e., was awake, had not had deteriorating neurologic function, had good protective reflexes, had not ingested a hydrocarbon, caustic, or strychnine), he was an excellent candidate for ipecac. We do not lavage if we can induce emesis since gastric recovery is almost complete with induced emesis, whereas lavage tubes will reliably and consistently miss much of the ingestant, especially if conglomerated. If we get no result by 25 minutes, we will repeat the ipecac dose (15 mL) plus 10 to 15 mL/kg of water. Failure to induce emesis after a second interval of 25 minutes requires removal of ipecac and the ingestant by lavage. Of course all requirements of a protected airway (normal gag reflex) must be fulfilled, otherwise we intubate via the trachea first with cuff in place prior to lavage.

Any material extracted by induction or lavage should be submitted for toxicologic analysis.

An IV line is indicated because at this level of toxicity, coma and shock are complications, and a good life line is mandatory throughout the stabilization phase and admission. Normal saline was selected as the initial fluid in case shock intervened. It was held at KVO until further assessment was completed. There was no indication for immediate forced diuresis in this ingestion. We favor an angiocath and would try a No. 18 or No. 20. It is perfectly acceptable to get venous samples from this line.

Toxicologic screen confirms the suspected ingestant but may also identify other toxins (note this child had one prior episode of ingestion). The CBC gives baseline information but may also be used to confirm the toxic iron level, in that a WBC count in excess of 15,000/cu mm has about 95% specificity for toxic iron levels over 300 mg/dL. The GI hemorrhage associated with significant iron intoxication may lead to hemorrhagic shock, so serial hematocrits should be obtained and a type and crossmatch sent. Serum electrolytes and ABGs may indicate the evolution of an anion-gap metabolic acidosis, associated with severe iron intoxication.

Children who do not develop GI symptoms of vomiting (usually bloody), abdominal pain (severe), or diarrhea (also bloody) by 6 hours post ingestion have not sustained serious degrees of iron intoxication, and this finding is necessary to release the child home after an adequate 6-hour observation. The child in this case has already manifested GI symptoms (pain and vomiting) and must be considered intoxicated.

Initial deferoxamine (Desferal®) IM injection can help ascertain that serum iron level is in excess of iron-binding capacity (the urine will turn ''vin rose'' color by 2 hours) and also acts as the initial therapy while iron levels and other determinants are being sought.

If the initial dose of deferoxamine is selected at 40 mg/kg, given IM, this will allow for a valid challenge, and yet not infringe on the maximum dosage allowable (generally 90 mg/kg every 8 hours) so that if the child decompensates, or has high initial levels, additional deferoxamine can be given IM. Remember that deferoxamine can be given intravenously only if the child is hypotensive. Limits on hourly IV infusion are usually 10 to 15 mg/kg/hr, so if the child becomes hypotensive during the course of IM therapy then the IV dosage rate must be adjusted for what was given already by the IM route. Unfortunately in the shock state, the IM absorption of medicine will be erratic.

Activated charcoal does not bind iron and is worthless in the management of isolated iron ingestion. We do not routinely use cathartics in toxic ingestions at our institution; this is a very controversial subject.

The x-ray may very well show radiopaque material in the stomach, and this would necessitate continued efforts to evacuate the stomach from above. This may entail repeated ipecac or Ewald lavage. Some centers recommend gastrotomy for retained iron.

Finally, all ingestions in our department are considered child neglect until proven otherwise, and a "SCAN" (Suspected Child Abuse/Neglect) consultation is obtained. This team approach usually involves a general pediatrician, an expert in abuse, and a social worker familiar with child protective services, abuse reporting, and crisis intervention for the family.

Lastly, the child is admitted to the intensive care unit where therapy with deferoxamine, as well as all aspects of medical and social support, can be continued.

SUGGESTED READINGS

Bachrach LL, Correa A, Levin R, et al: Complications of hypertonic phosphate lavage—iron poisoning. *J Pediatr* 1979;4:147.

LaCouture PG, Wason S, Temple AR, et al: Iron overdosage—emergency assessment of severity by laboratory methods. *J Pediatr* 1981;99:89.

Robertson WO: Iron poisoning—a problem of childhood. In Bager MJ, Rumack BM (eds): *Topics in Emergency Medicine*. Rockville, MD, Aspen Systems Corporation, 1979, pp 57–63.

Three-and-one-half-year-old Male with Wheezing, Cyanosis, and Fever

CASE PRESENTATION

A 3½-year-old male presented to the emergency department with a 2-day history of difficulty breathing that had become progressively worse. He was well until 7 days prior to presentation when he developed a runny nose and cough. Initially, the discharge was clear, but it has turned thick and green. He developed a fever 2 days prior to presentation. His mother noted that he was wheezing yesterday and has had progressively more trouble breathing. He has had one previous episode of wheezing that was treated with orally administered metaproterenol. His mother gave him a dose of the metaproterenol about 6 hours prior to presentation. He has never been admitted or required corticosteroids. There is a strong family history of asthma and allergies. There is no known history suggestive of a foreign body aspiration, tuberculosis, or cardiac disease. The child has had no medications except metaproterenol and acetaminophen (Tylenol®). He was eating well until today. His immunizations are up to date. His past medical history and review of systems are otherwise noncontributory.

Vital Signs

HR: 150 beats/min
RR: 45/min
T: 38.6°C (101.5°F)
BP: 105/70 mm Hg (expiration) and 95/70 mm Hg (inspiration)
WT: 17 kg
HT: 90 cm
M²: 0.7

Physical Examination

GEN: Slightly lethargic child, sitting upright with circumoral cyanosis

HEENT: *Head:* NCAT. *Eyes:* clear conjunctiva; tears; EOM intact; PERRLA; flat discs. *Ears:* clear tympanic membranes. *Nose:* thick green discharge from nares. *Oropharynx:* clear with moist mucous membranes

NECK: Supple with trachea midline; no crepitance on palpation, no stridor

CHEST: Suprasternal and intercostal retractions; breath sounds diminished bilaterally but are symmetric; diffuse expiratory wheezes and rales; inspiratory/expiratory ratio of 1:3

CVS: Tachycardia without S_3, S_4, or murmur; full pulses

ABD: Normoactive bowel sounds; no hepatosplenomegaly, masses, or tenderness

EXT: No bony or joint abnormalities

NEURO: Slightly lethargic; results of cranial nerve, motor, sensory, and coordination examinations grossly normal

SKIN: Circumoral cyanosis

SUGGESTED INTERVENTIONS

1. Administer oxygen, 6 L/min, via nasal prongs.
2. Administer epinephrine, 1:1,000 dilution, at a dose of 0.17 mL SC.
3. Place on cardiac monitor.
4. Suction if necessary.
5. If no improvement after 20 minutes, give second dose of epinephrine, 0.17 mL, 1:000, SC.
6. If still no improvement after another 20-minute interval, give nebulized metaproterenol, 0.2 mL diluted in 3 mL normal saline.
7. Failure to respond to three interventions defines "status asthmaticus." Establish an IV line and give 102 mg (6 mg/kg) of aminophylline over 20 to 30 minutes; then place on a continuous infusion consisting of 5% dextrose in 0.45 normal saline to run at 105 mL/hr (one and one-half times maintenance) plus aminophylline, 17 mg/hr (1 mg/kg/hr).
8. Obtain blood specimens for ABGs, CBC, and blood culture and sensitivity.
9. Give methylprednisolone sodium succinate (Solu-Medrol®), 35 mg (2 mg/kg), IV bolus.
10. Order chest x-ray (portable).
11. Admit to ICU.

CASE DISCUSSION

Asthma is very common in the pediatric population. It is a leading cause of school absences and visits to emergency departments. Each year it is the cause of

100 to 200 deaths. To avoid unnecessary morbidity and mortality the clinical evaluation of the patient's status, diagnosis, and institution of therapy must be done quickly and decisively.

A patient such as the one in this case study with a previous history of wheezing does not pose a difficult diagnostic dilemma. The most difficult case is the young child or infant with his first episode of wheezing. For the infant under 2 years with a history of upper respiratory tract symptoms and fever preceding the onset of wheezing, bronchiolitis secondary to respiratory syncytial virus or parainfluenza virus would be a likely diagnosis. It is difficult to tell, however, if this represents the first episode of wheezing in what will prove to be an asthmatic child. Some studies suggest that a respiratory syncytial virus infection may predispose the child to asthma. The wheezing of bronchiolitis may or may not be responsive to bronchodilators. A test dose of epinephrine, 1:1,000, at a dose of 0.01 mL/kg with a maximum of 0.35 mL or metaproterenol aerosol treatment may be given to determine if the patient is responsive to bronchodilators.

Also the differential diagnosis of wheezing must include foreign body aspiration. Often the wheezing is asymmetric. In addition, there is usually a history of choking and coughing. The diagnosis may depend, however, on a high index of suspicion. Inspiration/expiration chest x-rays, including left and right decubitis films, or fluoroscopy may aid in the detection of foreign body aspiration, by revealing "mediastinal swing," air trapping, and/or a fixed diaphragm on the side of the aspiration.

Pneumonia of any etiology (viral, bacterial, mycoplasmal, or tubercular) may be associated with wheezing. This wheezing may or may not be responsive to bronchodilator therapy. At times, especially in young children, it may be difficult to distinguish wheezing from the transmitted upper airway noises associated with an upper respiratory tract infection, croup, epiglottitis, retropharyngeal abscess, and so on. A careful physical examination with comparison of peripheral breath sounds to auscultatory findings over the trachea may aid in making the distinction. Pulmonary edema associated with myocardial failure may be associated with wheezing (cardiac asthma). Again, the physical examination for the presence of jugular venous distention, gallop rhythm, murmur, hepatomegaly, or peripheral edema will be helpful. The distinction is important because in congestive heart failure therapy with epinephrine may be highly detrimental.

There are several important aspects of the history that will aid in the treatment of patients with asthma. Questions should be directed at determining the duration of the wheezing and any antecedent illnesses. Sinusitis, for instance, causes an exacerbation of asthma but is poorly responsive to bronchodilator therapy until the sinusitis is aggressively treated. This child has a history that is suggestive of sinusitis with a long duration of upper respiratory tract symptoms, purulent nasal discharge, and onset of fever. The history of the course of the child's previous episodes of wheezing and response to therapy will aid in determining whether ICU care is likely. The child's current medications, including the last theophylline dose, will, in part, determine whether a theophylline level is needed prior to bolusing or starting a maintenance theophylline drip. The number and timing of recent emergency department visits is also important. A child who has had two to three visits to the emergency department in the past 24 hours warrants admission to the hospital.

The initial priority on physical examination is to evaluate the severity of the illness and respiratory distress. The patient may range from normal to agitated to stuporous, since hypoxia and hypercapnia supervene. With increasing respiratory effort the patient may assume an upright sitting position, and intercostal, sub-costal, and suprasternal retraction may be apparent as the patient uses the accessory muscles of respiration. Circumoral cyanosis and acrocyanosis may be difficult to detect. Often the child appears mildly dehydrated secondary to decreased intake and increased insensible losses. The respiratory rate and heart rate are usually elevated. An elevated temperature suggests infection or atelectasis. Pulsus paradoxus, if present, indicates severe airway obstruction. Normally during inspiration there is decreased left-sided cardiac filling with a concomitant fall in systolic blood pressure. A decrease of greater than 10 mm Hg is abnormal and indicates severe airway obstruction. Crepitance palpated in the neck and supraclavicular areas is suggestive of a pneumothorax or pneumomediastinum. A shift of the trachea from the midline is suggestive of a tension pneumothorax. Auscultation of the chest is important to assess ventilation. Expiratory wheezing and a prolonged expiratory phase are common in mildly to moderately severely affected children. As the severity of the obstruction increases the chest may actually become quieter with decreased breath sounds and decreased wheezing. Very asymmetric breath sounds with an absence in one hemithorax should raise the suspicion of a pneumothorax or major lobar atelectasis. Rales and rhonchi may be heard in patients with asthma without a pneumonia being present. Diaphoresis, lethargy, and fatigue are all signs of impending respiratory failure. This child appeared moderately distressed with decreased responsiveness, pulsus paradoxus, cyanosis, and evidence of maximal respiratory effort. There was no evidence of pneumothorax.

An ABG analysis is essential to assess ventilation in all but mildly affected asthmatics. The results, however, must be interpreted together with the clinical evaluation. A Pco_2 of 40 mm Hg in a child with retractions and tachypnea is a sign of severe obstruction since hypocarbia would be expected in a patient expending that much respiratory effort. Sequential blood gas determinations are important in following the moderate to severe asthmatic. A rising Pco_2 is a sign of worsening obstruction and/or fatigue. This patient's ABGs were pH, 7.36; Po_2, 90 mm Hg; and Pco_2, 36 mm Hg. Even a Pco_2 approaching a normal of 40 mm Hg is a "danger signal" of impending fatigue and failure.

A CBC obtained after giving epinephrine will typically have an elevated WBC count. It may, however, be important to obtain a hemoglobin and hematocrit in a child with moderate to severe asthma in order to evaluate the oxygen-carrying capacity. A blood culture is indicated in the toxic-appearing febrile child. Unless a pneumothorax is suspected, radiographic studies can usually wait until the patient has stabilized. A chest x-ray will show signs of air trapping with hyperinflation and flattened diaphragms. Atelectasis, pneumonia, pneumomediastinum, and pneumothorax all may be uncovered. Further studies should be done as indicated. This patient has a history suggestive of sinusitis so a sinus series should be obtained once the patient stabilizes.

Oxygen should be started on all patients who are more than mildly affected. The patient immediately "pinked" up after receiving oxygen. In general there are no contraindications to the use of oxygen in children even if there is a long history of asthma. The initial approach to β-adrenergic drug administration varies from physician to physician. Some use nebulization and others subcutaneous administration as their initial intervention. The most common approach is to begin, as was done with this patient, with subcutaneous administration of epinephrine. The dose is 0.01 mL/kg of the 1:1,000 dilution up to a maximum of 0.35 mL SC. This can be repeated every 20 minutes to a maximum of three doses. The use of epinephrine is contraindicated if the patient has received a series of injections within the previous 6 hours. Studies suggest that the third of three doses of epinephrine provides no more therapeutic advantage than just two doses of epinephrine. In view of this, a nebulized β-adrenergic agent may be more efficacious as the second or third intervention. Commonly used nebulized β-adrenergics include isoetharine and metaproterenol. The latter has fewer cardiac side effects. The usual doses of nebulized metaproterenol are 0.1 mL in children under 2 years old, 0.2 mL in those aged 3 to 7 years, and 0.3 mL for children over 7 years of age. The dose is mixed with 3 mL of normal saline, and the entire volume is given. Intermittent positive-pressure breathing (IPPB) is contraindicated for children. In general, a patient who continues to wheeze, to have diminished peak flows, or to have any distress after the third intervention should be admitted. Peak expiratory flow rate (PEFR) is difficult to measure in children under 5 years of age or in any patient who is severely distressed. When able, we like to evaluate and document the PEFR before and after therapy. A standard for discharge from the emergency department is a PEFR equal to or greater than 65% of expected PEFR. A "ballpark" formula to calculate expected PEFR is shown below:

$$\text{Males: } 6 \, (HT_{cm}) - 500 = PEFR$$
$$\text{Females: } 5 \, (HT_{cm}) - 400 = PEFR$$

In addition, those patients who are dehydrated, have had two or more emergency department visits in the previous 24 hours, or have parents unable to cope with their illness should also be admitted.

Patients who have not been on a theophylline preparation prior to presentation and are scheduled for admission should be bolused with 6 mg/kg Aminophylline® (lean body weight) IV over 20 to 30 minutes and then started on a maintenance drip of aminophylline of 1 mg/kg/hour. The dose for the maintenance drip will need to be lowered for patients under 1 year of age and over 14 to 16 years of age. The goal of therapy is to achieve a level between 12 to 15 μg/dL. Patients who are on a short-acting preparation and who have not had a dose for greater than 6 hours should be bolused and started on a maintenance drip as above. Patients who are on a short-acting preparation who have had a dose within the past 6 hours should have a theophylline level drawn and a maintenance drip begun. The bolus should await the theophylline level results. Patients who are on long-acting theophylline preparations and have had a dose within the previous 6 hours should have a theophylline level drawn. The bolus and maintenance administration should await the result of the level. Patients who are on a long-acting theophylline preparation but who have not had a dose in the previous 6 hours should also have a theophylline level drawn. In these patients a maintenance aminophylline drip is indicated, but the bolus should await the results of the level. The loading dose or bolus of aminophylline to be given once the peak blood theophylline level is known can be calculated from the formula (15 − theophylline level)/2. A dose of 1 mg/kg will raise the serum level by 2 μg/dL. If the level is greater than or equal to 13 μg/dL, then no bolus is necessary.

The subject is still somewhat controversial, but probably all children who are admitted for asthma should be started on corticosteroid therapy. Methylprednisolone sodium succinate (Solu-Medrol®), at a dose of 2 to 3 mg/kg IV given initially and every 6 hours, will avoid some of the mineralocorticoid effects seen with hydrocortisone sodium succinate (Solu-Cortef®). Improvement should start within 6 to 8 hours after the initiation of corticosteroid therapy. Sedatives are contraindicated. Often these children are mildly dehydrated. Total fluids at one to one and one-half times maintenance are usually sufficient. In the very severe rare case of asthma with increasing P_{CO_2} despite aminophylline, corticosteroids, and nebulized therapy, IV therapy with isoproterenol (Isuprel®), intubation, and mechanical ventilation may be required. The dosage range for IV infusion of isoproterenol is 0.05 to 0.50 μg/kg/min.

All patients with asthmatic status should be admitted to a pediatric intensive care unit.

The patient in this case study was admitted to the pediatric ICU. He remained on IV therapy with aminophylline for 36 hours and then was transferred to the ward, where he was switched to an oral long-acting theophylline preparation, prednisone, and metaproterenol. He was discharged on day 4 of admission to continue the oral therapy with prednisone for a total of 5 days, the theophylline for 2 weeks, and the metaproterenol for 2 weeks and then on an as needed basis.

Follow-up with a pediatrician or family practitioner was stressed in view of the chronic nature of asthma. He was given a 2-week course of ampicillin for sinusitis.

SUGGESTED READINGS

Burowsky M, Nakatsu K, Munt P: Theophylline reassessed. *Ann Intern Med* 1984;10:63.

Rachelefsky G, Katz R, Siegel S: Chronic sinus disease associated with reactive airway disease in children. *Pediatrics* 1984;73:526.

Stempel D, Mellon M: Management of acute severe asthma. *Pediatr Clin North Am* 1984;31:879.

Case 31

Four-year-old Male with Cystic Fibrosis

CASE PRESENTATION

A 4-year-old white male was diagnosed with cystic fibrosis at the age of 9 months. He presented to the emergency department with a 1-week history of increasing cough and wheezing and high fevers. Today he has had difficulty catching his breath and appears "bluer than normal" to his mother. His last admission in the hospital was 5 months ago for 2 weeks for pneumonia. He is followed monthly in the cystic fibrosis clinic. His regular medications are Pancrease®, Fer-In-Sol®, multivitamins, and vitamin E and A supplements.

Vital Signs

T: 38.5°C (101.3°F)
HR: 150 beats/min
RR: 65/min
BP: 95/70 mm Hg
WT: 15 kg

Physical Examination

GEN: Thin, pale white acrocyanotic male in moderate respiratory distress and 5% to 10% dehydrated
HEENT: *Nose:* clear nasal rhinitis. *Oropharynx:* 2+ enlarged tonsils without exudates; dry mucous membranes
NECK: Supple with anterior cervical adenopathy; nontender

CHEST: Bilateral rhonchi, wheezes, and rales; breath sounds greater on the right than left; accessory muscles used; intracostal and supraclavicular retractions evident
CVS: Regular rate and rhythm without murmurs, lifts, or gallop rhythms
ABD: Soft; benign; normal bowel sounds
GU: Normal Tanner stage I male, uncircumcised
EXT: Clubbing and cyanosis in all extremities

SUGGESTED INTERVENTIONS

1. Administer oxygen, 4 to 5 L/min, via mask or nasal prongs.
2. Start IV line with normal saline. Administer bolus, 20 mL/kg (300 mL) then at 1½ maintenance (80 mL/hr) pending laboratory results.
3. Order blood specimens for ABGs, CBC, blood culture, and electrolytes. Dextrostix® (result = 80 mg/dL).
4. Administer aminophylline, 90-mg bolus over 15 minutes, then 15 mg/hr continuous infusion.
5. Administer ticarcillin 750 (50 mg/kg, IVSD) and tobramycin, 22 mg (1.5 mg/kg, IM).
6. Order chest x-ray (portable, upright, full expiration).
7. Admit the patient (preferably to a regional cystic fibrosis center).

CASE DISCUSSION

Cystic fibrosis is the most common lethal genetic disease of childhood and adolescence. It has autosomal recessive transmission and occurs once in 1,800 births. The prevalence in the United States is 1:33,000, and about 1,500 new cases are diagnosed each year. It occurs predominantly in whites but is seen in blacks and orientals as well. It was first described as a unique disease entity in the 1930s. At that time the life expectancy was only a few years; now it is 25 to 30 years of age, with a few patients living into their late 40s. The average age of diagnosis is 4 to 6 months, but because of wide variability of expression of the disease and improper diagnosis, some cases are not identified until their teens and 20s.

The above case study is typical of a young child with cystic fibrosis deteriorating as pneumonia develops. The suggested interventions will evaluate the respiratory and metabolic status of the child, relieve the distress caused by hypoxia, and rule in or out the possibility of pneumonia, atelectasis, or pneumothorax. The WBC count is often elevated to 10,000 to 20,000/cu mm. ABG determinations might show hypoxia and hypercarbia, but this should be compared with the child's baseline studies to determine the severity of his current condition. The ABGs might also show a metabolic alkalosis. Sodium and chloride levels may be decreased, especially in hot weather when a child with cystic fibrosis loses large amounts of these electrolytes in his sweat. The chest x-ray might show hyperinflation, pneumothorax, atelectasis, infiltrates, increased bronchovascular markings, or cyst formation. This should also be compared with previous films if available. Fluid replacement is important, not only for the dehydration, but also for pulmonary function by helping to mobilize the thick tenacious mucus in the lungs. Pneumothorax is uncommon in a patient this young. If greater than 10%, it should be treated with needle aspiration and then, if persistent, with thoracostomy drainage. Extreme caution should be taken not to cause a larger pneumothorax since the pulmonary status in these patients is often tenuous. Oxygen therapy can make the patient more comfortable, but it should not be so high (i.e., greater than $FIo_2 = 40\%$) as to suppress the hypoxic respiratory drive.

Cystic fibrosis is a disease that affects every organ system, but primarily the respiratory and GI systems. The basic defect is mucoviscoidosis (i.e. abnormally thick secretions) of the exocrine glands. Studies point to a defect in the specialized epithelial cells lining the exocrine glands. Chloride ions are not able to cross cell membranes, causing electrolyte and fluid abnormalities within the glands. The genetic and biochemical defects have not been identified yet, and there is no cure. Some patients are sick from infancy and die at an early age. Others have a more benign course and lead relatively healthy lives until their 20s and 30s. Early diagnosis and initiation of treatment enhances life expectancy.

The lungs are slowly and irreversibly damaged by the thick bronchial secretions. The normal ciliary cleaning activity and host defenses are impaired, leading to chronic infections. Initially, *Staphylococcus aureus* predominates; later it is mostly *Pseudomonas*. Pneumococcus, *Hemophilus influenzae, Proteus, Escherichia coli,* and *Klebsiella* are also found. The chronic infections and secretions lead to alveolar and bronchial obstruction, hyperinflation, atelectasis, scarring, and formation of cavities. Bronchospasm is commonly seen, appearing similar to asthma. Empyema, pneumothorax, and pneumomediastinum are seen in later years. Hemoptysis, caused when large cavities erode into bronchial vessels, can be fatal in the end stages of cystic fibrosis. Chronic hypoxia and pulmonary hypertension eventually lead to cor pulmonale and congestive heart failure.

The GI tract is affected as thick secretions in the pancreatic ducts prevent normal secretion of the digestive enzymes trypsin, lipase, and amylase into the duodenum. This leads to malabsorption of food and passage of frequent bulky foul-smelling stools. Inadequate uptake of nutrients, especially proteins, essential fatty acids, fat-soluble vitamins, and minerals can lead to severe malnutrition, even to pellagra and kwashiorkor. In some patients the pancreas is so destroyed that it loses its endocrine function as well and diabetes mellitus ensues. The biliary ducts can also become obstructed by thick secretions, leading to portal hypertension, hypersplenism, bleeding varices, cirrhosis of the liver, and ascites.

The sweat glands of the skin produce large amounts of sweat with a high sodium and chloride content, causing the characteristic "salty taste" of a person with cystic fibrosis. This can lead to heat prostration with lethargy, abdominal pains, vomiting, and shock on very hot days.

Other complaints of cystic fibrosis include clubbing of the digits, nasal polyps, sinusitis, rectal prolapse, bleeding disorders, growth retardation, inguinal hernia, scoliosis, osteoporosis, delayed sexual maturation, amenorrhea, sterility and infertility, bowel obstruction, brain abscess, osteomyelitis, cheilosis, anemia or polycythemia, gynecomastia, adrenal failure, anosmia, night blindness, and many others. The psychological toll of chronic illness and frequent hospitalization, school absenteeism, short stature, and a cachectic appearance can be devastating on a child or an adolescent.

The diagnosis of cystic fibrosis is made by clinical findings and a sweat chloride determination (positive if greater than 60 mEq/L in a sweat sample weighing 50 mg or more). There is a potential for prenatal diagnosis of cystic fibrosis. Fetal α-phosphatase in the amniotic fluid is very low in 90% of those who will develop cystic fibrosis. Neonatal screening of serum trypsin by immunoreactive assay (increased in cystic fibrosis) has potential for earlier detection of the disease.

The basis of therapy is early, frequent, and aggressive nutritional and antibiotic treatment. High-protein, high-caloric diets with vitamin and mineral supplements are stressed, along with pancreatic enzyme replacement (Viokase®, Cotazyme®, and Pancrease®). Antibiotics are used almost continuously in some centers. Oral, IV, and aerosolized routes are employed. Many variations are tried, most commonly the combination of an aminoglycoside (tobramycin or gentamicin) with an anti-*Pseudomonas* penicillin (ticarcillin or pipericillin). Vigorous chest physiotherapy is used from infancy onward. Theophylline and aerosolized water are also used. Patients with cor pulmonale can benefit from digitalis preparations and diuretics.

The emergency department physician can also look for undiagnosed cystic fibrosis. Patients with chronic cough, chronic bronchitis or pneumonia, atypical or resistant asthma, failure to thrive, unexplained malnutrition, chronic diarrhea or steatorrhea, salty taste, or nasal polyps should be referred for a sweat chloride test.

Virtually all patients with cystic fibrosis presenting to the emergency department warrant serious consideration for admission, no matter what their presentation. Admission to a regional cystic fibrosis center is recommended.

SUGGESTED READINGS

Arehart-Treichel J: Cystic fibrosis linked to chloride ions' inability to cross certain cells, and Cystic fibrosis research looks promising. *JAMA* 1985;252:2519.

Cystic Fibrosis: A Summary of Symptoms, Diagnosis and Treatment. Rockville, MD, Cystic Fibrosis Foundation, 1979.

di Sant'Agnese P: Cystic fibrosis. In *Nelson's Textbook of Pediatrics.* Philadelphia, WB Saunders, 1979, pp 1988–2001.

Moss AJ: The cardiovascular system in cystic fibrosis. *Pediatrics* 1982;70:728.

Porter DK, Van Every MJ, Anthracite RF et al: Massive hemoptysis in cystic fibrosis. *Arch Intern Med* 1983;143:287.

Schwachman H: Cystic fibrosis. *Curr Probl Pediatr* 1978;3:10.

Taussig LM, Landau LI: Cystic fibrosis. In Kelley VC (ed): *Practice of Pediatrics*. Philadelphia, Harper & Row, 1981.

Four-year-old Female with Abdominal Pain, Vomiting, and Lethargy

---

CASE PRESENTATION

A 4-year-old female presented with a 1-day history of abdominal pain, vomiting, and lethargy. There was no diarrhea, constipation, dysuria, fever, toxic ingestion, or trauma. The pain was diffuse and constant. She had vomited six times in the past 24 hours. Emesis was nonbilious. Until the day of presentation she had been eating very well. She had had a 6-pound weight loss over the past 3 weeks. She had a 2-week history of polyuria and polydipsia. She had received no medications. The past medical history was significant for chickenpox 2 months previous to arrival in the emergency department.

Vital Signs

HR: 128 beats/min
BP: 95/60 mm Hg
RR: 38/min
T: 37.4°C (99.3°F)
WT: 14 kg
HT: 101 cm

Physical Examination

GEN: Thin female with deep respirations
HEENT: *Head:* atraumatic. *Eyes:* sunken, clear conjunctiva; PERRLA; EOM intact; flat discs with no retinal changes. *Oropharynx:* dry mucous membranes; marked odor of acetone on breath

NECK: Supple, no thyromegaly or adenopathy

CHEST: Deep respirations without retractions; otherwise clear to percussion and auscultation

CVS: Sinus tachycardia without S_3, S_4, or murmur; normal pulses

ABD: Hypoactive bowel sounds; liver 1 cm below right costal margin; normal spleen; no masses; diffuse tenderness without localization, guarding, or rebound; no costovertebral angle tenderness

GU: *Rectum:* normal tone, heme − stool

EXT: No clubbing, edema, or cyanosis

NEURO: Slightly lethargic, but easily arousable, oriented, and cooperative; intact cranial nerves II through XII; normal motor and sensory examination, coordination, and reflexes

SKIN: Dry, but no tenting; fair peripheral perfusion

SUGGESTED INTERVENTIONS

1. Administer oxygen, 3 L, via nasal prongs.
2. Place on cardiac monitor with rhythm strip.
3. Take postural vital signs.
4. Start IV line with 0.45 normal saline to run at 800 mL every 8 hours plus potassium chloride, 15 mEq, every 8 hours.
5. Obtain blood specimens for Chemstrip® (over 400 mg/dL), electrolytes, BUN, glucose, CBC, phosphate, venous pH, and serum acetone.
6. Obtain urine sample for sugar and acetone and complete urinalysis (3 + sugar, large ketones).
7. Give regular insulin mixed as 50 units in 250 mL normal saline to run at 1.4 units/hr, which equals 7 mL/hr.
8. Order Chemstrip® or glucose determination every hour.
9. Admit patient for hydration, insulin, and diabetic education.

CASE DISCUSSION

Diabetic ketoacidosis is the most common cause of altered mental status and acidosis in children. Only about 30% of new-onset type I diabetics present in frank ketoacidosis. The majority of new diabetics will present with the classic history of polyuria, polydipsia, polyphagia, and weight loss. Another common complaint is diffuse abdominal pain with emesis secondary to ketosis and hypokalemia, with ileus and decreased blood flow to the splanchnic vessels. Frequently there is lethargy secondary to dehydration and hyperosmolarity. Deep Kussmaul respirations, with a fruity or acetone breath, represent an attempted respiratory compensation for the metabolic acidosis. In children, concurrent infections such as candidiasis or pyogenic skin infections are rare, although a leukocytosis is common.

Since the most significant morbidity and mortality in the treatment of childhood diabetic ketoacidosis is caused by cerebral edema secondary to rapid changes in osmolarity, careful attention must be paid to correction of the fluid and electrolyte imbalances. At presentation in diabetic ketoacidosis most patients are 7% to 10% dehydrated. Changes in vital signs including posturals should be used to assess the extent of dehydration. Unless the patient is at least 7% to 10% dehydrated there is no need to bolus fluids. When boluses are required, 10 to 20 mL/kg of normal saline can be given over 30 to 60 minutes. Replacement of the water deficit should be accomplished over 30 to 36 hours. The replacement volume plus maintenance fluids should not exceed 4,000 mL/M^2 or 4,000 mL, whichever is least, over a 24-hour period, in order to avoid cerebral edema. If the serum glucose value is greater than 300 mg/dL, the fluids should be given as 0.45 normal saline. If the serum glucose value is less than 300 mg/dL, fluids should be given as 5% dextrose in 0.45 normal saline. Fluids may need to be increased to keep up with urinary losses secondary to glycosuria.

Children with poorly controlled diabetes of long standing may present with hyponatremia. The hyponatremia may be fictitious secondary to lipidemia, or it may represent a total body sodium depletion secondary to natriuresis. The sodium deficit is calculated as (135 − patient's volume) × (0.6) × (patient's weight in kilograms) to be corrected over 24 hours. Hyperchloremia resulting from fluids with a sodium concentration greater than 0.45 normal saline may prolong the acidosis, and overcorrection of the sodium deficit will increase the hyperosmolarity.

The most serious electrolyte disturbance is potassium depletion. An ECG may provide rapid evidence of hypokalemia or hyperkalemia. Potassium chloride at a dosage of 3 mEq/kg/24 hr should be added to the initial IV fluids if there are no ECG changes of hyperkalemia, the initial potassium value is less than 6 mEq/L, and there is no history of anuria. If there is ECG evidence of hypokalemia, flattened T waves or presence of U waves, or an initial serum potassium value of less than 3 mEq/L, potassium chloride at a dosage of 4 to 8 mEq/kg/24 hr should be added to the initial IV fluids. In the presence of acidosis a normal serum potassium value represents a total body potassium deficit. Potassium is drawn into the extracellular space as hydrogen ions are drawn to the intracellular space to be buffered. Potassium should be monitored frequently since both the resolution of the acidosis and the treatment with insulin will precipitate movement of potassium into the intracellular space, leading to hypokalemia.

In the majority of cases the acidosis will respond to hydration and insulin therapy alone. Sodium bicarbonate, especially when used as a bolus, can cause a paradoxic CNS acidosis resulting in alterations in cerebral blood flow, cerebral edema, and coma. Carbon dioxide is the by-product of the reaction, $HCO_3^- +$

$H^+ \rightarrow H_2CO_3 \rightarrow H_2O + CO_2$, and more easily diffuses across the blood–brain barrier than $HCO_3{}^-$. In addition, $NaHCO_3$ may overcorrect the acidosis, precipitating hypokalemia. Elevation of the serum sodium value also contributes further to the hyperosmolarity. Current recommendations suggest that $NaHCO_3$ should be used only if the serum pH is less than 7.1, *and* the serum bicarbonate level is less than 10 mEq/L. It should not be given as a rapid or bolus infusion but rather as a continuous infusion of 1 mEq/kg over 4 to 8 hours. The serum potassium value should be monitored closely during the infusion. The infusion should be discontinued when the serum pH reaches 7.2.

Insulin may be administered in several ways. Because of the ease of control, low-dose continuous infusion of regular insulin intravenously at a dose of 0.1 unit/kg/hr is recommended. Fifty units of regular insulin U-100 is mixed with 250 mL of normal saline to yield a concentration of 1 unit/5 mL. An initial bolus of insulin has not been found to promote more rapid control. Blood glucose levels must be monitored hourly. When the glucose level falls below 300 mg/dL, 5% dextrose should be added to the IV fluids. When the glucose level falls below 200 mg/dL, 10% dextrose should be added to the IV fluids. Insulin may be given subcutaneously at doses of 0.3 to 2 units/kg every 4 to 6 hours. To prevent cerebral edema, the serum glucose value should drop at a maximum rate of 100 mg/dL/hr and should not be allowed to drop below 150 mg/dL in the first 24 hours of therapy.

The use of phosphate remains controversial and has not been shown to decrease the morbidity or mortality of childhood diabetic ketoacidosis. The use of excessive amounts of phosphate may precipitate hypocalcemia. Some centers recommend alternating potassium chloride and potassium phosphate in the IV fluids to not only correct the phosphate deficit but also to avoid hyperchloremia.

Admission is indicated for correction of dehydration and electrolyte imbalances and for insulin therapy. For the well-known diabetic with recurrent ketoacidosis, treatment in an emergency department setting may be appropriate, but all patients with new-onset diabetes should be admitted not only for medical therapy but also for intensive education.

SUGGESTED READINGS

Duck SC, Weldon VV: Cerebral edema complicating therapy for ketoacidosis. *Diabetes* 1976;25:111.

Foster D, McGarry JD: The metabolic derangements and treatment of diabetic ketoacidosis. *N Engl J Med* 1983;309:159.

Kaplan S: *Clinical Pediatric and Adolescent Endocrinology.* Philadelphia, WB Saunders, 1982, pp 131-156.

Kaufman I, Keller M, Nyhan W: Diabetic ketosis and acidoses: The continuous infusion of low doses of insulin. *J Pediatr* 1975;87:846.

Kaye D: The bicarbonate controversy. *J Pediatr* 1973;87:156.

Perkin R, Marks J: Low dose continuous intravenous insulin infusion in childhood diabetic ketoacidosis. *Clin Pediatr* 1979;18:540.

Case 33

Four-year-old Male with Ingestion of Liquid Drain Cleaner

CASE PRESENTATION

A 4-year-old male presented 1 hour after ingesting an unknown amount of a liquid drain cleaner containing sodium hydroxide and sodium hypochlorite. The mother was cleaning the bathroom sink when the ingestion took place. The child splattered some of the cleaner on his clothes. After the ingestion the mother gave the child 5 ounces of milk. There is no history of emesis, respiratory distress, pain, or watering of eyes. There is no previous history of ingestion of foreign substances, broken bones, or burns. The mother could not identify any recent life stresses. The medical history was otherwise noncontributory. Immunizations are up to date.

Vital Signs

HR: 110 beats/min
RR: 24/min
BP: 90/60 mm Hg
T: 37°C (98.6°F)
WT: 18 kg

Physical Examination

GEN: Well-developed male with wet clothing
HEENT: *Head:* NCAT. *Eyes:* right conjunctiva injected; EOM intact; PERRLA; flat discs; vision, 20/20. *Ears:* normal tympanic membranes. *Nose:* nares normal. *Oropharynx:* injection of the soft palate, but no ulcers; swollen lower lip; drooling

NECK: Supple
CHEST: *Lungs:* No retractions, clear to percussion and auscultation
CVS: Regular rate and rhythm without S_3, S_4, or murmur; full pulses
ABD: Normoactive bowel sounds; no tenderness, masses, or hepato-
        splenomegaly
GU: Normal prepubertal male
EXT: No bony or joint abnormalities
NEURO: Grossly normal

SUGGESTED INTERVENTIONS

1. Keep patient NPO.
2. Keep patient in upright sitting position.
3. Irrigate each eye with 1 L of normal saline. Check pH in conjunctival sac at end of lavage.
4. Remove soiled clothes and rinse skin with water until the soapy sensation has disappeared.
5. Request ophthalmology consultation.
6. Request otolaryngology consultation.
7. Begin IV of 5% dextrose in 0.2 normal saline to run at 55 mL/hr with potassium chloride, 18 mEq/24 hr.
8. Obtain blood specimen for CBC.
9. Order chest x-ray.
10. Admit patient for endoscopy and observation.

CASE DISCUSSION

Alkalis such as sodium hydroxide (lye), sodium hypochlorite (bleach), and ammonium hydroxide are commonly found in household cleaners. Ingestion of corrosives represent 1% to 2% of all accidental ingestions, with 90% of the ingestions involving children under 5 years of age. The majority of the ingestions of household cleaners occur in the home while the product is in use. The Food and Drug Administration now requires that products with concentrations greater than 10% of corrosives be packaged in childproof containers. Most household bleaches contain sodium hypochlorite in dilute concentrations and do not represent a risk. Most serious ingestions involve dishwasher detergents or lye (sodium hydroxide, potassium hydroxide) found in oven cleaners, drain cleaners, and Clinitest® tablets.

Alkalis may cause burns when they come in contact with the eyes, skin, oropharynx, GI tract, and respiratory tract. Alkalis, especially lye, can penetrate deeply into tissues, causing liquefaction necrosis and thrombosis of vessels, leading to further ischemia. This destruction is enhanced by the release of heat. The acute necrosis and inflammation is maximal at about 1 week. Acute complications include perforation of viscera. With healing, scar tissue formation leads to strictures of the esophagus and/or stomach, with 80% of strictures becoming symptomatic in the first 2 months after ingestion.

The majority of children present with a history of an observed ingestion. Acutely, the child may present to the emergency department with drooling, dysphagia, abdominal pain, or refusal to eat secondary to burns of the oropharynx, esophagus, or stomach. The oropharynx needs to be carefully examined for injection and ulcers; however, the absence of lesions in the oropharynx does not rule out lesions in the esophagus or stomach. In children, crystal alkaline products may be expectorated so that only oropharyngeal lesions will be present. With liquids there is a higher probability that the alkali will be swallowed, resulting in lesions of the stomach and esophagus. There may be evidence of respiratory distress secondary to inhalation of fumes or glottic edema. Contact with the skin may also cause burns. Caustics cause rapid and devastating damage to the eyes, ranging from mild irritation to complete necrosis of the cornea in a few minutes.

The basics of life support—airway, breathing, and circulation (the ABCs)— should be evaluated especially for signs of respiratory distress. Commonly, bleach and drain cleaners are erroneously mixed with cleanser, generating chlorine and chloramine gases. After assessing the ABCs, any possible exposure to the eyes should be treated immediately with copious irrigation for at least 20 minutes with water. Alkalis penetrate very deeply. If after irrigation the pH of the tears tested with litmus paper is greater than 7.7, irrigation should be continued. An ophthalmologist should be consulted as soon as possible. Contaminated clothing should be removed and the skin rinsed with water until the soapy feeling is gone.

Some authors advocate giving milk, 15 mL/kg, with a maximum of 240 mL in order to dilute the alkali and decrease the exothermic activity. Volumes greater than this are contraindicated to prevent gastric distention and emesis. All fluids should be withheld if there is any evidence of respiratory distress, difficulty handling secretions, or planned endoscopy or surgery under anesthesia. Emesis should not be induced in order to prevent further mucosal damage. Giving weak acids to neutralize the alkali is contraindicated because of the resulting exothermic activity. The child should be kept in an upright sitting position to prevent reflux and aspiration. An otolaryngologist should be consulted as soon as possible. Endoscopy is indicated if the child is symptomatic or there are oropharyngeal lesions. If endoscopy is to be performed, the child should be kept NPO and a maintenance IV started. If the child is asymptomatic and there are no oropharyngeal lesions the otolaryngologist may elect to admit the child and observe. If endoscopy is to be performed, usually it is done within 24 hours of the exposure to decrease the risks of perforation. If there are any signs or symptoms of esophageal or gastric perforation, chest and upright abdomen films are indicated.

Passage of an NG tube has not been shown to prevent the development of strictures and may cause emesis or perforation. Corticosteroids have been shown to be beneficial for moderate burns but should not be started until consultation is obtained. Prophylactic antibiotics are not indicated unless there has been perforation.

About 25% of children will be involved in more than one ingestion. A prominent risk factor for childhood ingestions of foreign substances is the degree of stress within the family. A social service consultation and possible family counseling should be considered for all episodes of childhood poisoning.

SUGGESTED READINGS

Hawkins D, Demeter M, Barnett T: Caustic ingestions: Controversies in management: A review of 214 cases. *Laryngoscope* 1980;90:98.

Henretig F, Cupit G, Temple A: Toxicologic emergencies. In Fleisher G, Ludwig S (eds): *Textbook of Pediatric Emergency Medicine*. Baltimore, Williams & Wilkins, 1983.

Moorhead J: Corrosive ingestions. In Bayer M, Rumack B, Wanke L (eds): *Toxicologic Emergencies*. Bowie, MD, Robert J. Brady Co, 1984.

Case 34

Four-year-old Male with Weakness, Tachycardia, and Palpitations

CASE PRESENTATION

A 4-year-old white male weighing 18 kg presented with a 4-hour history of fatigue, nausea, tachypnea, and palpitations, specifically a "fluttering" in the chest. The child's mother stated he had seemed pale and diaphoretic for the last hour or so.

The patient had not been ill with the exception of a mild afebrile upper respiratory illness 1 week prior to presentation. He has been afebrile, there has been no vomiting, and oral intake was normal on the day of presentation.

On close questioning the mother does recall two similar episodes of palpitation that resolved spontaneously in 4 to 6 hours. There is no history of chest pain, syncope, cyanosis, or family history of heart disease. The patient has never had an ECG performed and is taking no medications.

Vital Signs

T: 36.8°C (98.2°F)
P: 210 beats/min
RR: 40/min
BP: 100/60 mm Hg

Physical Examination

GEN: Well-developed, well-nourished, pale and diaphoretic male who is slightly short of breath but is alert, conversant, and ambulatory
HEENT: Normal results of examination; no perioral cyanosis

NECK: Supple without adenopathy; no neck vein distention, no stridor; midline trachea; no hepatojugular reflex (HJR)

CHEST: Clear to auscultation and percussion; no rales or dullness to percussion at bases; mild subcostal retractions

CVS: Regular rapid rhythm; regular S_1 and S_2; no murmur; examiner unable to appreciate a gallop rhythm; quiet precordium; point of maximal impulse in left fourth intercostal space in the midclavicular line

ABD: No organomegaly; soft; nontender; normal bowel sounds without ascites

EXT: Pulses rapid but good quality; no edema; no cyanosis

NEURO: Alert; active; normal motor, sensory, and cranial nerve reflexes; examination oriented

SUGGESTED INTERVENTIONS

1. Administer oxygen, 3 L/min, via nasal prongs.
2. Order ECG with 12- or (13-) lead ECG and rhythm strip.
3. Place patient on continuous cardiac monitoring.
4. Establish IV line with normal saline or lactated Ringer's KVO.
5. Test vagal maneuvers: Valsalva, carotid massage; perform rectal examination; have patient cough; check diving reflex (ice and water in plastic bag, to patient's face). If unsuccessful . . .
6. Administer verapamil, 0.1 mg/kg, IV over 30 seconds; may repeat dose once in 5 to 15 minutes. Have calcium chloride 10% on hand.
7. Admit or refer. Discuss case with pediatric cardiologist.

CASE DISCUSSION

The case presented here in many respects represents a very straightforward case of paroxysmal atrial tachycardia (PAT). The diagnosis of PAT can be made electrocardiographically by the presence of a rapid ventricular rate (e.g., 200 beats/min) with narrow QRS complexes indicating impulse formation "above" the level of the ventricles. P waves are frequently not seen, although this is not a requirement. The rhythm is occasionally associated with Wolff-Parkinson-White syndrome, but ECG findings of this syndrome are not seen in the tachyarrhythmic phase, owing to anterograde conduction down normal pathways with retrograde conduction via the accessory pathways. This illustrates the reentrant mechanism of SVT. It is frequently impossible to determine the electrophysiologic etiology of an SVT rhythm in the emergency setting.

Aside from the entity of recurrent PAT, there are two more common clinical presentations. The first is acute onset of SVT without failure. This usually occurs in children over 1 year of age, such as in the case presented. This presentation responds well to vagal maneuvers or therapy with verapamil.

The second common presentation occurs in the infant who frequently is under 4 months of age. These patients typically present with hypotension and in heart failure. In a large study in 1981, 38% of infants with PAT who were under 18 months of age were in overt congestive heart failure. This poses a significant diagnostic challenge to the emergency department physician. Although PAT has been called the most common dysrhythmia of childhood, it is quite uncommon, with an incidence of 1 in 25,000 reported in 1967. The number of infants presenting with shock and sinus tachycardia from noncardiogenic sources far exceeds this, with dehydration and sepsis the leading etiologies. Treatment of these entities with verapamil can have serious adverse consequences. The onus is on the emergency department physician to diagnose the cause of shock. Instituting cardioversion or antiarrhythmic agents in these cases may further decrease cardiac output.

Cardioversion beginning at 0.25 to 0.5 J/kg is the treatment of choice for a patient determined to have PAT who presents with severe failure or hypotension in these patients. It is inappropriate and time consuming to attempt lengthy vagal maneuvers. The electrical discharge should be synchronized to avoid R on T phenomenon. Digitalization at 40 to 50 μg/kg (total digitalizing dose) should be carried out after successful cardioversion, as in adults; giving digoxin prior to cardioversion is discouraged because of increased arrhythmogenicity and risk of ventricular fibrillation following cardioversion. Patients with ectopic pacemakers (a less common phenomenon) are less likely to respond to cardioversion; their ventricular rate may be slowed, however, by blocking conduction with digoxin.

Vagal maneuvers are least effective in small infants but work well in older children. The diving reflex is the most likely vagal maneuver to be effective in infants. To perform it correctly, ice and water should be placed in a bag or rubber glove and held tightly (so as to make respiration difficult) over the infant's nose and mouth for 20 to 45 seconds. Less aggressive approaches are likely to fail. Eye pressure is not recommended in pediatric patients.

Verapamil has come to be the pharmacologic treatment of choice in all pediatric patients over 2 years of age with SVT. Recent studies show excellent response to verapamil in pediatric patients whose SVT is secondary to reentry. It has compared favorably with propranolol (Inderal®) and digoxin for long-term control. Care must be taken to avoid its use when a condition other than SVT exists and when decreased cardiac output would be hazardous. It should be used with caution, if at all, when propranolol, quinidine, or disopyramide (Norpace®) are in use concurrently. As in adults, it is considered dangerous in patients who have Wolff-Parkinson-White syndrome with a past history or present occurrence of atrial fibrillation. The correct pediatric dosage is 0.1 mg/kg IV over 1 to 2 minutes. It may be repeated in 30 minutes. Hypotensive response to this calcium-channel blocker should be reversed with calcium chloride, 10%, 0.2 mL/kg, slow IVp.

Alternate choices to verapamil include phenylephrine and propranolol. Edrophonium (Tensilon®) is used only rarely in childhood and is dangerous. Phenylephrine is a nice choice when the child is initially only slightly hypotensive (10% reduction in systolic pressure or less). The dosage is 0.01 mg/kg and is repeated as needed. The systolic blood pressure must be monitored. Conversion frequently occurs as the blood pressure rises, and vagal maneuvers should be repeated during this phase; they work better in normotensive patients. Propranolol is effective when verapamil is contraindicated. These two drugs, both negative inotropes, should not be used together or in sequence. Propranolol is relatively contraindicated in congestive heart failure (unless the heart failure is directly rate related), bronchospastic diseases, and diabetes, the last primarily because β-blockade masks the signs of hypoglycemia, so if Dextrostix® results are followed, the drug could be used safely. One popular dosing regimen for propranolol in this setting is 0.01 to 0.02 mg/kg, IV, every 10 to 15 minutes until conversion is achieved, to a maximum dosage of 0.1 mg/kg.

Admission criteria for patients with SVT are straightforward. A patient in severe congestive heart failure or cardiogenic shock who cannot be converted by countershock needs admission to an ICU.

Any patient successfully cardioverted in the emergency department should be digitalized as an inpatient and requires at least a monitored bed. Any patient who requires acute digitalization should be admitted. Patients who correct with verapamil or vagal maneuvers and who did not present with distress may be discharged on no medications presuming adequate follow-up. Arguably these patients should stay on oral "maintenance" therapy with verapamil, but this has not yet been established in the pediatric population. Patients with refractory, asymptomatic SVT who do not convert (usually older patient with chronic SVT) can be sent home provided they, their parents, and the physician to whom they are referred are comfortable with this decision.

Propranolol certainly plays a role in the treatment of refractory or recurrent SVT. Presuming one followed the protocol described here, however, verapamil would have been used first, and the use of the two drugs simultaneously is contraindicated.

This child failed to respond to vagal maneuvers but converted immediately with verapamil. He had brief sinus bradycardia but quickly stabilized with normal sinus rhythm, with normal blood pressure and relief of symptoms.

Repeated 12-lead ECGs showed classic type "A" Wolff-Parkinson-White syndrome, with preexcitation and delta waves.

This patient went home on maintenance therapy with verapamil, on the advice of the staff "on-call" pediatric cardiologist.

SUGGESTED READINGS

Garson A, Gillette PC, McNamara DG, et al: Supraventricular tachycardia in children: Clinical features, response to treatment, and long term follow-up in 217 patients. *J Pediatr* 1981;98:875.

Gillette PC, Adams D: Dysrhythmias. In Adams (ed): *Moss' Heart Disease in Infants, Children, and Adolescents,* ed 3. Baltimore, Williams & Wilkins, 1983.

Porter CT, Gillette PC, Garson A, et al: Effects of verapamil on supraventricular tachycardia in children. *Am J Cardiol* 1981;48:487.

Sapire DW, O'Riordan AC, Black IF: Safety and efficacy of short- and long-term verapamil therapy in children with tachycardia. *Am J Cardiol* 1981;48:1091.

Winniford M, Fulton KL, Hillis LD: Long-term therapy of paroxysmal supraventricular tachycardia: A randomized, double-blind comparison of digoxin, propranolol, and verapamil. *Am J Cardiol* 1984;54:1138.

Four-year-old Male with Fever, Rash, and Swollen Extremities

CASE PRESENTATION

A 4-year-old Asian male presented with a 5-day history of fever. He was well until 5 days ago when he developed a spiking temperature to 40°C (104°F). One day after onset of the fever he developed a red rash over his extremities and trunk. Three days after onset of the fever he developed painful swelling of his hands and feet. He had been seen by his pediatrician 2 days after onset of the fever with the diagnosis of a viral syndrome. He has no runny nose, cough, diarrhea, abdominal pain, sore throat, or vomiting. He has continued to take fluids well, and urine output has been normal. His mother became concerned because he seemed to be breathing faster. There is no history of recent camping or travel. There are no household pets or standing water. There is no history of ingestions of foreign substances. His immunizations are up to date, including a mumps/measles/rubella at age 15 months. He has never had an episode of fever, rash, or swelling. He has been on no medications except aspirin.

Vital Signs

HR: 145 beats/min (regular)
RR: 35/min
T: 40°C (104°F)
BP: 95/60 mm Hg
WT: 18 kg

195

Physical Examination

GEN: Alert, well-developed male in mild respiratory distress

HEENT: *Head:* NCAT. *Eyes:* conjunctiva bilaterally injected with no exudate; PERRLA; EOM intact; flat discs. *Ears:* tympanic membranes erythematous but mobile. *Nose:* clear nares. *Oropharynx:* injected, but with no exudate; lips red and cracked

NECK: Supple; isolated, enlarged, right anterior cervical node measuring 1.5 cm; no jugular venous distention

CHEST: 1+ retractions with bibasilar rales; good air exchange

CVS: Tachycardia with S_3 and S_4; heart sounds are not muffled; no murmur; full pulses

ABD: Soft; normal bowel sounds; no masses or tenderness; liver 2 cm below right costal margin

GU: Normal male

EXT: Hard, nonpitting edema of the hands and feet plus palmar erythema

NEURO: Alert and grossly normal

SKIN: Diffuse erythematous, raised rash with large, irregularly shaped plaques; no cyanosis with capillary refill of less than 3 seconds

SUGGESTED INTERVENTIONS

1. Administer oxygen, 5 L/min via nasal prongs.
2. Place on cardiac monitor and obtain 12-lead ECG.
3. Establish an IV line with 5% dextrose in water and run at KVO.
4. Obtain blood specimens for CBC and platelet count, blood culture, ABGs, ESR, electrolytes, SGOT, SGPT, and streptozyme. Dextrostix® (result = 80 µg/dL).
5. Order urinalysis and throat culture.
6. Perform chest x-ray.
7. Administer furosemide (Lasix®), 1 mg/kg, IV or IM.
8. Request consultation of a pediatric cardiologist and infectious disease or rheumatology specialist.
9. Begin therapy with aspirin, 100 mg/kg/day, divided into four doses.
10. Admit for close observation, 2D-echocardiography, possible digitalization, immune serum globulin, anti-inflammatory therapy, and further workup.

CASE DISCUSSION

Kawasaki's disease (mucocutaneous lymph node syndrome) is a relatively newly described syndrome. The signs and symptoms in the acute phase may mimic many other infectious and rheumatologic diseases so that the diagnosis may be difficult and a high index of suspicion is required. Establishing the diagnosis is critical because of the high incidence of cardiac complications (20%) and the risk of sudden death.

Kawasaki's disease occurs in all races, but its incidence is highest among orientals of Japanese ancestry. Eighty percent of cases are reported in children under 4 years old. It occurs not only in sporadic cases but also in limited epidemic outbreaks.

The etiology of the disease is unknown. No infectious agent has been identified so far. It is associated with certain HLA types, suggesting a genetic predisposition. Circulating immune complexes have been found to be elevated, but the pathophysiologic significance remains unclear. The major pathologic findings are a progressive vasculitis with a predilection for the coronary arteries and other small- and medium-sized arteries.

Kawasaki's disease is characterized by fever, rash, conjunctivitis, mucous membrane lesions, edema, and lymphadenopathy. The major diagnostic criteria are listed below with at least five of the features required to make the diagnosis. Since the disease evolves over time, all the features may not be apparent at the time the child presents to the emergency department.

Fever for more than 5 days
Conjunctival injection
Changes in the mouth: erythema, fissuring, and crusting of lips; diffuse
    oropharyngeal erythema; strawberry tongue
Changes in the peripheral extremities: induration of hands and feet; erythema of
    palms and soles; desquamation of tips and fingers and toes 2 weeks from
    onset of illness
Erythematous rash
Lymphadenopathy with at least one lymph node mass more than 1.5 cm in
    diameter
No evidence for other systemic illness

Kawasaki's disease progresses through three phases. The acute phase (7 to 14 days) is characterized by fever, conjunctival injection, rash, swelling of the hands and feet, oral lesions, and lymphadenopathy. The subacute phase begins with resolution of the rash and fever and is characterized by arthritis, irritability, thrombocytosis, desquamation, myocarditis, development of aneurysms, and coronary thrombosis. During this phase, which lasts 4 to 6 weeks, the risk of death is highest. The last phase, convalescent, lasts up to 2 years and is characterized by the resolution of symptoms and aneurysms.

The fever begins abruptly and heralds the onset of the illness. It commonly reaches 40°C (104°F) with multiple spikes per day. It persists 1 to 4 weeks.

Bilateral conjunctival injection without exudate usually begins 2 days after the onset of the fever and persists 1 to 5 weeks. It occurs in 96% of cases. Corneal ulcers do not usually occur, although uveitis has been described.

Mucous membrane changes occur in 99% of cases and include injection of the oropharynx, erythema and fissuring of the lips, and hypertrophic papillae of the tongue (strawberry tongue). These changes usually occur within 1 to 3 days after the onset of fever. Mucosal ulcers and a sore throat are rare, although soreness of the lips is common.

Characteristic extremity changes (erythema of the palms and soles, edema of the hands or feet, and peripheral desquamation) occur in 99% of cases. The swelling and erythema usually begin within 3 days of the onset of the fever. The edema is firm and indurative without pitting. The child may refuse to walk or use his hands secondary to pain. The skin on the hands and feet begins to peel around the nails 2 to 3 weeks after the onset of the fever.

A rash is seen in 99% of cases and begins soon after the onset of the fever. It characteristically is pruritic and occurs in large, raised, irregular, red plaques over the trunk and extremities. Less frequently it may be maculopapular or even mimic erythema marginatum.

Cervical adenopathy occurs in 82% of cases. The most common presentation is a single nonsuppurative, firm, enlarged node of more than 1.5 cm in diameter. The adenopathy usually appears within 3 days after onset of the fever and lasts 1 to 3 weeks.

Pyuria secondary to a urethritis with no renal involvement occurs in 75% of cases. Arthralgias and arthritis of primarily the large joints occurs in 35% to 45% of cases. Sleep disorders and irritability are common. Aseptic meningitis may be present in 25% of cases during the acute phase. Gastrointestinal disturbances such as abdominal pain and diarrhea may be present in another 25% of cases. Ten percent of patients have hepatitis, and 5% have hydrops of the gallbladder suggested by a right upper quadrant mass.

Cardiac complications are the most important pathologic changes found in the 2% of the patients who die of Kawasaki's disease. Less than 5% of the fatalities occur during the acute phase, while 70% of the deaths occur between 15 and 45 days after onset of the fever (i.e., subacute phase). During the acute phase the pathologic findings of the heart include a perivasculitis of the coronary arteries, microvascular angiitis, pericarditis, and inflammation of the atrioventricular conduction system. Coronary aneurysms are found 12 to 28 days after onset of the fever while myocardial and endocardial inflammation is decreasing. Clinically in the first week a severe tachycardia out of proportion to the fever may be seen. The more serious abnormalities such as congestive heart failure, pericardial effusions, and arrhythmias secondary to a pancarditis are usually seen 9 to 21 days after the fever. However, as in this patient, they may occur earlier. Symptoms and signs of cardiac involvement include irritability, vomiting, decreased peripheral perfusion, tachycardia, a gallop rhythm, tachypnea, rales, hepatomegaly, and edema. Distended neck veins, a narrowed pulse pressure, tachycardia, and congestive heart failure, if present, are suggestive of a pericardial effusion with impending tamponade. The chest x-ray may show cardiomegaly and pulmonary edema. In patients with cardiac involvement the ECG usually shows heart block, PR interval prolongation, ST-T wave changes, and voltage changes. Decreased contractility, pericardial effusion, and coronary aneurysms are well seen on a 2D-echocardiogram. The majority of deaths are secondary to thrombosis of coronary aneurysms during the subacute phase of the illness leading to myocardial infarction. This should be suspected in the child who experiences an acute decompensation in hemodynamic status.

This patient, although in the acute phase, has clinical evidence of cardiac dysfunction. The gallop rhythm, rales, hepatomegaly, and tachypnea are suggestive of congestive heart failure secondary to myocarditis. The absence of jugular venous distention, narrowed pulse pressure, or muffled heart sounds is evidence against a significant pericardial effusion. The onset early in the course argues against thrombosis of a coronary vessel and myocardial infarction as the cause of the congestive heart failure.

Essential to the diagnosis of Kawasaki's disease is the exclusion of diseases that may mimic the syndrome. A careful history of exposure, travel, and the sequence of the symptoms and signs is important. Of particular concern are the infectious diseases that require immediate antibiotic therapy to prevent increased morbidity and mortality. It may be necessary to administer appropriate antibiotics until the diagnosis of Kawasaki's disease can be confirmed. Kawasaki's disease may mimic streptococcal scarlet fever and sepsis, although less than 5% of patients have a scarlatiniform rash. Laboratory evidence of a streptococcal infection such as a throat culture or positive streptozyme may be helpful. Toxic shock syndrome and staphylococcal scalded skin syndrome may also be in the differential diagnosis. However, the rash of Kawasaki's disease is rarely pustular, and if present the shock associated with Kawasaki's disease is more likely to be cardiogenic rather than septic. Culture evidence of a staphylococcal infection or colonization may be confirmatory. Serum calcium levels and hematocrits are reliably depressed in the majority of patients with toxic shock syndrome. Leptospirosis is also in the differential diagnosis. A history of exposure to animals or standing water as well as laboratory confirmation with titers will be helpful. Rickettsial diseases such as Rocky Mountain spotted fever must be considered especially since cardiac dysfunction may be prominent to both. However, Rocky Mountain spotted fever is characterized by a hemorrhagic dependent rash, thrombocytopenia, and disseminated intravascular coagulation. Measles, rubella, and Epstein-Barr virus infections may also mimic Kawasaki's disease. Measles and rubella would be rare in the immunized patient. Epstein-Barr infections can be confirmed by titers or heterophile slide test.

One noninfectious disease in the differential diagnosis is the Stevens-Johnson syndrome. The lack of an offending drug and the absence of mucosal and conjunctival ulcerations may be helpful in ruling out this syndrome. The collagen vascular diseases such as scleroderma, systemic lupus erythematosus, and juvenile rheumatoid arthritis may mimic Kawasaki's disease. The marked elevation of the sedimentation rate seen in these rheumatologic conditions is not seen in Kawasaki's disease. Again, laboratory evaluation and subsequent chronicity of symptoms will aid in the diagnosis. Rheumatic fever should be considered; however, strict adherence to Jones criteria with evidence of a prior streptococcal infection will confirm the diagnosis. Blacks are overrepresented in the population of Kawasaki's disease patients. In the young black child presenting with swollen hands and feet a sickle screen should be obtained to rule out hand-and-foot disease. This patient's history and results of physical examination are very suggestive of Kawasaki's disease, and another etiology would be very unlikely.

Laboratory tests are not diagnostic of Kawasaki's disease. The WBC count is usually elevated with a predominance of neutrophils. The sedimentation rate and C-reactive protein uniformly rise during the acute phase of the disease and then decline during the subacute phase. Thrombocytosis is seen in almost all cases, with the increase beginning about 10 days after onset of the fever and correlating with the peak incidence of coronary thrombosis. A blood culture is indicated to help rule out infections such as *Streptococcus* or *Staphylococcus*. A streptozyme and throat culture may also help. Liver enzymes, prothrombin time, and bilirubin determinations should be obtained not only for evidence of hepatitis but also as a baseline for subsequent aspirin therapy. In a patient such as this one who presents with signs and symptoms of cardiac dysfunction, an ABG is required, as are baseline electrolyte values in anticipation of diuretic therapy and possible digitalization. Further blood work, such as leptospirosis titers, should be based on the history and clinical picture. A urinalysis will show a sterile pyuria in 75% of cases. A chest x-ray and ECG are mandatory on presentation, not only as evidence of cardiac dysfunction but also to serve as a baseline. A 2D-echocardiogram should be obtained in all patients. Angiography will be indicated in only a small portion of the patients.

Most children with Kawasaki's disease should be admitted to a hospital. For children with clinical, radiographic, or ECG evidence of cardiac disease, admission is mandatory. Consultation with a pediatric cardiologist and infectious disease or rheumatology specialist should be obtained. All patients sent home with Kawasaki's disease require initial biweekly follow-up. Currently therapy is mostly supportive. Aspirin is used in the acute phase for its anti-inflammatory properties and chronically for its antiplatelet properties. During the acute phase it is administered at a dosage of 100 mg/kg/day divided into four doses. Levels are monitored to prevent toxicity. After resolution of the fever, the dose is decreased to 10 mg/kg/day. Other antiplatelet therapy such as dipyridamole may be used when aneurysms are present. γ-Globulin therapy during the acute phase is being investigated, and initial results are promising. In patients such as this one who has evidence of cardiac dysfunction, again the care is primarily supportive. Oxygen should be administered. The treatment of the congestive heart failure includes diuretics and inotropic agents such as digitalis, dopamine, and dobutamine. Digitalization in the patient with myocarditis needs to be done carefully and under the supervision of a cardiologist.

Follow-up is essential. Most of the aneurysms will resolve within 6 months. The exact risks for subsequent angina and sudden death in the future for these patients is still under investigation. For the majority of patients it is a self-limited disease.

This patient was started on aspirin, furosemide, immune serum globulin, and digoxin at a dose of 12 μg/kg/day. A 2D-echocardiogram done on admission showed evidence of decreased ventricular contractility but no effusion. He responded well to therapy, with his fever resolving in 10 days. A repeat echocardiogram on day 15 showed an aneurysm of the left anterior descending coronary artery. He was maintained on low-dose aspirin therapy, and the aneurysm had resolved on a follow-up echocardiogram done after 12 months. He continues to do well with no sequelae.

SUGGESTED READINGS

Bell DM, Morens DM, Holman RC, et al: Kawasaki syndrome in the United States. *Am J Dis Child* 1983;137:211.

Burns JC, Glode MP, Clarke SH, et al: Coagulopathy and platelet activation in Kawasaki syndrome: Identification of patients at high risk for development of coronary artery aneurysms. *J Pediatr* 1984;105:206.

Fujiwara H, Hamashima Y: Pathology of the heart in Kawasaki disease. *Pediatrics* 1978;61:100.

Lapointe N, Chad Z, LaCroix J, et al: Kawasaki disease: Association with uveitis in seven patients. *Pediatrics* 1982;69:376.

Melish M, Hicks R, Reddy V: Kawasaki syndrome: An update. *Hosp Pract* 1982;17:99.

Novelli VM, Galbraith A, Robinson PJ, et al: Cardiovascular abnormalities in Kawasaki disease. *Arch Dis Child* 1984;59:405.

Slovis TL, Hight DW, Phillipart AI, et al: Sonography in the diagnosis and management of hydrops of the gallbladder in children with mucocutaneous lymph node syndrome. *Pediatrics* 1980;65:789.

Case 36

Four-year-old Female with Vaginal Discharge

CASE PRESENTATION

A 4-year-old white female was brought to the emergency department because of a persistent greenish vaginal discharge. This discharge had been present for several months despite careful cleaning of the vaginal area and use of several emolient creams. The child was finally brought to medical care because she had begun to complain of dysuria. The mother had noted on multiple occasions that the child was manipulating or scratching her perianal area. The mother stated that the child wore cotton panties and did not use bubble bath.

Prior medical history revealed that the child had a normal birth and perinatal period. She was fully immunized and had no past serious illnesses or hospitalizations. There were no drug allergies.

Family history revealed an 8-year-old sister and a 1-year-old half-sister. The mother was 30 years of age. The 35-year-old natural father had not seen the child in more than 3 years. A stepfather, age 38, resided with the family. The child does not attend preschool or day care. The mother is employed as an assembly line worker. The stepfather is intermittently employed.

Vital Signs

HR: 95 beats/min
RR: 18/min
BP: 86/55 mm Hg
T: 37.6°C (99.6°F)
WT: 16 kg

Physical Examination

HEENT: Normal examination
NECK: Shotty nodes
CHEST: Clear
CVS: Regular; no murmur
ABD: Soft; nontender; normal bowel sounds; no organomegaly or masses
GU: *Vagina:* obvious greenish white discharge at the introitus; hymenal opening of 10 mm with old transection at 6 o'clock; scar along the midline raphe from the posterior fourchette toward the anus. *Rectum:* hypertrophy of the anal folds and several scars from old tears radiating out from the anal opening at 5 and 7 o'clock; touching the anus with a finger led to gaping of the structure
NEURO: Walked normally and spoke in full sentences

SUGGESTED INTERVENTIONS

1. Prepare the child for vaginal examination.
2. Order gonorrheal, chlamydial, and routine cultures of the vaginal discharge, including slide fluorescent antibody test for *Chlamydia*.
3. Order wet mount, potassium hydroxide, and Gram stain of the vaginal discharge.
4. Order gonorrheal cultures of throat and rectum.
5. Order VDRL.
6. Treat suspected gonorrhea with amoxicillin, 50 mg/kg, plus probenecid, 25 mg/kg (maximum, 1 g) given concurrently.
7. Request immediate social service consultation to interview the child.
8. Notify child protective agency and police.
9. Complete appropriate reporting forms.
10. Place patient and her siblings in foster care.
11. Make appointments for medical follow-up of cultures and psychologic evaluation and support.

CASE DISCUSSION

Until 1978, child sexual abuse was barely discussed, let alone recognized. Since that time there has been a rapid advance in the understanding and diagnosis of child sexual abuse. At present it is estimated that 60% of all females are sexually misused in some manner by the age of 18 years. Sexual abuse of male children is less frequently reported, but there is increasing concern that similar numbers of boys are also abused.

The abusers are usually known to the family. In fact, only 7% of the time is the assailant unknown to the child and family. Child sexual abuse cases generally arrive in the emergency department because the possibility of abuse has arisen. However, as sophistication increases, more children are recognized as abused just on physical findings alone.

Once the possibility of abuse exists the child should be interviewed alone by a professional skilled in talking with children. The interviewer wants to determine who, what, where, when, and how the abuse took place. The following general comments can be made about the history in cases of child sexual abuse. The abuser rarely hurts the child but rather slowly escalates the degree of invasiveness. The mean time from onset of abuse to reporting is currently 3½ years. The abuser uses gifts, threats, and/or establishment of a "secret between us," to prevent the child from reporting the abuse. Additionally, the children usually have intense, albeit irrational, guilt feelings surrounding the abuse. Therefore, great care is needed to reassure the child that it is okay to talk about these events. The child should be asked to indicate as much as possible exactly what events took place. The use of anatomically correct dolls facilitates the interview in very young children.

The following physical findings are compatible with child sexual abuse:

Acute Recent Abuse

1. Vaginal
   a. Bruising or small lacerations around the introitus or of the hymen
   b. New laceration of posterior fourchette
   c. Erythema of hymen or vaginal walls
   d. Sexual abuse creates injuries generally from 3 to 9 o'clock; straddle injuries produce findings at 12 and 6 o'clock.

2. Rectal (examination except for observation may be deferred if the child is very tender)
   a. Perianal contusion
   b. Fresh fissures
   c. Edema of rectal wall
   d. Anal spasm
   e. Rectal ampulla lacerations (rare)

Chronic

1. Vaginal
   a. Multiple hymenal transection between 8 and 4 o'clock
   b. Rounded hymenal remnants
   c. Scar or scars at 6 o'clock position in posterior fourchette

    d. Gaping spacious introitus

    e. Hymenal opening greater than 4 to 5 mm up to 5 years of age, 10 mm 5 to 10 years of age, and 15 mm at puberty

    f. Synechia between hymen and vaginal walls or synechia on hymen indicating healing of a hymenal transection

    g. Thickening of hymen

2. Rectal

    a. Often no injuries because lubricant and slow penetration are used

    b. Hypertrophy of folds

    c. Submucous thickening

    d. Gaping of anus when touched, lax sphincter tone

    e. Scars from old anal tears

The usual forensic examination and collection of evidence in acute cases of rape rarely apply to child sexual abuse. However, in cases of acute abuse the appropriate portions of the adult forensic examination should be done. This will include looking for dried semen as well as aspirating the vagina with a small plastic catheter. A speculum examination is not necessary in cases of child sexual abuse unless a foreign body is suspected or there is concern about major trauma to the vagina or rectum. In these cases examination under anesthesia should be done. A rectal examination and x-ray film may help determine the need for examination with anesthesia.

Venereal diseases in children, as in adults, are transmitted sexually. Condylomata and herpetic lesions are very suggestive of sexual contact unless the child had a wart or herpetic lesion elsewhere on the body predating the vaginal appearance. Cultures for *Chlamydia* should always be obtained. However, the significance of this organism is still being debated. If chlamydial infection is diagnosed it should be treated with erythromycin, not tetracycline, in order to avoid permanent dental stains.

The presence of intracellular gram-negative diplococci on Gram stain of a vaginal discharge does not always indicate gonorrhea is present in prepubertal girls. Therefore, we do not make a definitive diagnosis based on the Gram stain, but we do prophylactically treat the child if the Gram stain indicates the possibility of gonorrhea.

All states have mandatory reporting laws and in most the report must be made immediately (orally) to the local child protective services. In this case the stepfather was identified as the abuser, and all the children were removed from the home pending court action.

Finally, it is important for the child protective services to get a complete written report of all findings on the appropriate reporting forms.

SUGGESTED READINGS

Cantwell HB: Vaginal inspection as it relates to child sexual abuse in girls under thirteen. *Child Abuse Neglect* 1983;7:171.

Felman YM, Nikitas JA: Sexually transmitted diseases and child sexual abuse. *NY State J Med* April 1979;79:714.

Goncalves-Teixeira WR: Hymenal colposcopic examination in sexual offenses. *Am J Forensic Med Pathol* 1981;2:209.

Josephson GW: The male rape victim: Evaluation and treatment. *JACEP* 1979;8:13.

Kramer DG, Jason J: Sexually abused children and sexually transmitted diseases. *Rev Infect Dis* 1982;4:588.

Neinstein JS, Goldenring J, Carpenter S: Nonsexual transmission of sexually transmitted diseases: An infrequent occurrence. *Pediatrics* 1984;74:67.

Orr DP, Prietto SV: Emergency management of sexually abused children. *Am J Dis Child* 1979;133:628.

Paul DM: The medical examination in sexual offenses against children. *Med Sci Law* 1977;17:251.

Rosenfeld AA: The clinical management of incest and sexual abuse of children. *JAMA* 1979;242:1761.

Woodling BS, Kossoris PD: Sexual misuse: Rape, molestation, and incest. *Pediatr Clin North Am* 1981;23:481.

Case 37

Five-year-old Female with Hypotension and Abdominal Pain

CASE PRESENTATION

A 5-year-old black female with known SS sickle cell anemia and many presentations to emergency departments for vaso-occlusive crises presented this time looking very pale, being short of breath, and complaining of severe abdominal pain.

She had upper respiratory tract symptoms for the past 3 days, characterized as a slight cough and congestion; she had only low-grade fever by the mother's observation. On the day of presentation she began to have severe abdominal pain, with a heaviness in her left upper quadrant. She became short of breath and then felt faint every time she stood up. Her mother, noting her almost passing out, brought her to the emergency department.

On her last visit to the emergency department 1 month previous, her hemoglobin value was 11 g/dL, and her reticulocyte count was 12%. She was admitted for simple vaso-occlusive crisis, requiring only modest analgesia and IV hydration. No major pulmonary, cerebral, or cardiac disease was detected. She was discharged on acetaminophen (Tylenol®) and folic acid therapy.

The past medical history revealed many visits for crises, that her immunizations were all current, and that she had received a Pneumovax® injection 2 years ago. There were no allergies, and she had had no operations. She had been maintained on a chronic transfusion program but discontinued it approximately 1 year previously because of the mother's objections.

Vital Signs

BP: 55 mm Hg (palpable)
P: 135 beats/min (weak and thready)

RR: 40/min (clear)
T: 38.4°C (101.1°F, rectal)
WT: 18 kg

Physical Examination

GEN: Well-developed, well-nourished black female, lying supine, in obvious distress

HEENT: *Eyes:* PERRLA; EOM intact; pale conjunctivae; flat fundi with "sickle" retinopathy. *Ears:* clear tympanic membranes. *Throat:* dry without enanthem

NECK: Supple; negative Kernig and Brudzinski signs; no nodes; no neck vein distention; no hepato-jugular reflex; midline trachea; no stridor

CHEST: Clear; increased respiratory rate; slight accessory muscle use; no nasal flaring; nontender chest wall; no pleural friction rub

CVS: Rapid regular rhythm, ?? summated gallop; + + murmur, grade III/VI; systolic flow type; no rub; no heaves; no lifts; normal P_2, increased S_1

ABD: Tender left upper quadrant mass, extending from left hypochondrium to left pelvic brim; normal bowel sounds; no rebound; no involuntary guarding; no hepatomegaly; no costovertebral angle tenderness

GU: *Rectum:* normal; nontender; heme-negative stool

EXT: Cool, clammy; no cyanosis, clubbing, or edema; all joints nontender and not enlarged; no extremity pain

NEURO: Alert; distressed; oriented to time, space, and self; normoreflexive; normal sensation

SUGGESTED INTERVENTIONS

1. Administer oxygen, 5 L/min, via nasal prongs.
2. Place on cardiac monitor.
3. Place in pediatric MAST suit, legs inflated. Put patient in Trendelenburg position.
4. Start 2 IV lines, large bore, normal saline; run in rapidly until blood pressure normalizes to systolic of 90 mm Hg.
5. Type and cross-match for 4 units packed RBCs. Ask specifically for sickle prep to be done on donor blood.
6. Order ABGs.
7. Order blood specimens for CBC, platelets count, blood culture, reticulocyte count, bilirubin, electrolytes, glucose, calcium, BUN, and creatinine.

8. Administer penicillin G, 50,000 units/kg IV, followed by ampicillin, 50 mg/kg, IV and chloramphenicol, 25 mg/kg IV.
9. Place Foley catheter for urimeter drainage; order stat urinalysis and urine culture and sensitivity.
10. Order chest x-ray (stat portable).
11. Institute partial exchange transfusion: 35 mL/kg of packed RBCs.
12. Admit the patient.

CASE DISCUSSION

The most rapidly fatal crises that a child with sickle cell anemia can sustain are overwhelming sepsis and splenic sequestration. The propensity for sicklers to develop infections with encapsulated organisms is well documented and most feared in the patient population under 2 years of age. This child was previously immunized with Pneumovax®, and this has shown to decrease the mortality somewhat; however, sepsis with pneumococci or other pathogens such as *Hemophilus influenzae* and enteric organisms is still possible. The slight elevation in temperature was suggestive of infection, but generally the sickler with sepsis classically has temperature over 39°C (102.2°F) or low temperature.

The rapid evolution of anemia, abdominal pain, and hypotension must be considered acute splenic sequestration until proven otherwise. In acute sequestration, blood is trapped in a rapidly enlarging spleen, leading to profound anemia and hypotension. Curiously, this serious complication occasionally follows minor upper respiratory tract type illnesses, as in this case. This condition particularly affects those with SC and S-β thalassemia to degrees and to ages past that which we expect it in SS disease. This child, however, was in the suspect age range for sequestration (i.e., 5 years of age or less). Sequestration over age 6 in SS disease is unusual but not unheard of.

The first consideration is reversing the hypovolemic shock. Exchange transfusion cannot be immediately instituted. Volume resuscitation must be done first. Oxygen is administered immediately, because of the shock, the compromised oxygen delivery, and anemia compounded by the dilution effect that will occur with the initial crystalloid infusion. Augmentation to IV volume infusion (which takes time to establish) includes the use of the pediatric MAST trousers and placing the patient in the Trendelenburg position. This will favor cerebral perfusion and help elevate peripheral resistance.

Cardiac monitoring will detect any arrhythmia, or cardiac ischemia, as well as indicate possible electrolyte abnormality.

The volume management in this seriously hypotensive child was to run in full-strength crystalloid (normal saline) until the blood pressure rose to her expected systolic level of 90 mm Hg. We use the patient's weight in kilograms added to 70 as an estimate of expected systolic pressure (in children over 1 year). With normalization of systolic blood pressure, the rate can be set down to 4 mL/kg/hr, and the child's vital signs watched meticulously for any secondary drop. This should prevent excessive hemodilution while partial exchange transfusion is being set up.

The type and cross-match should be for enough blood, in packed cell form, to accomplish a partial exchange transfusion of approximately 35 mL/kg. This would be 630 mL, so 3 units should suffice. It is wise to ask the laboratory to screen for sickle hemoglobin in the donor blood, since this is *not* routinely done in blood banking of donors.

Blood samples for ABGs were sent off to assess the degree of metabolic acidosis. This would be on the basis of poor perfusion and will always make sickling worse. Alkalinization can be done empirically with 1 mEq/kg infused and an additional 2 mEq/kg added to the next 4 hours worth of IV fluid, or it can be done on the basis of electrolytes, using the formula for base deficit:

$$\text{Bicarbonate deficit (mEq)} = (25 - HCO_3^-) \times 0.4 \times kg$$

This amount can then be administered in a fashion similar to that described above, with 1 mEq/kg IV initially and then the remainder over the next 4 hours. As in all patients with alkalinization, serum pH, serum potassium, and urine pH should be monitored.

The remaining laboratory tests were to be used to assess the possibility of infection as well as to compare hematologic values to past known results. The glucose, BUN, creatinine, and calcium values were all done as baseline and may be expected to change if exchange transfusion is instituted.

The hemoglobin returned was 2 g/dL, and the reticulocyte count was 50%. Platelets were 75,000/cu mm, which is a very common finding with sequestration. Thrombocytopenia usually corrects with reversal of the shock, as well as transfusion with fresh blood. The WBC count was 17,000/cu mm with left shift. Although this is consistent with infection, it is also highly characteristic of sequestration. The ESR is totally useless for the determination of sepsis in the actively sickling patient, and the use of C-reactive protein is not well studied.

Based on the suspicion of sepsis, antibiotics were pushed. The basis for this decision was temperature, hypotension, and elevated WBC count with shift. Although statistically unlikely, the mortality of untreated underlying bacteremia is so high that we elected to treat with antibiotics. The organisms most feared are pneumococci and *Hemophilus influenzae*. Accordingly, we elected to infuse penicillin G, 50,000 units/kg, IV as treatment for pneumococci and follow that with ampicillin and chloramphenicol, which would be continued intravenously during the admission. Cultures were performed prior to the push of antibiotics, with the exception of CSF fluid. Although there was no meningismus, and in general sickle cell patients over 1 year of age should show this finding with meningeal infection, there have been many classic reports of febrile patients with sickle hemoglobinopathies who do not show initial meningismus and then die of meningitis (usually pneumococcal). This child was too hemodynamically unstable to have a lumbar puncture done initially; after stabilization, performing a lumbar puncture in the emergency department could be reconsidered. It was not a serious omission to delay the spinal tap, as long as the antibiotics were used first.

A urinary catheter was placed to follow urine output, which is a must in any hypotensive patient. The urine indices in sicklers may be misleading in that with advancing age they lose the ability to concentrate urine and to retain sodium. So if the specific gravity is monitored to gauge the adequacy of the volume restoration, a serious error might be made. Instead, absolute outputs, state of hydration, perfusion, respiratory rate, and ABGs are followed. Similarly, a high urine sodium level does not mean the absence of volume depletion in these patients. Incidentally, sicklers tend to dehydrate hypotonically owing to this loss of sodium in excess of water.

Following all these resuscitative measures a portable anteroposterior chest x-ray was obtained. The purpose of this film is multifold. The presence or absence of pulmonary infiltration will help rule in or out the diagnosis of pneumonia infarction or pulmonary edema. The heart size will be very important in the speed and quantity of transfusion. Mild sequestration (*not* in this patient) can be managed with simple transfusion, in which case 10 mL/kg of packed RBCs is slowly infused over several hours to reverse the anemia and vascular compromise. In cases of manifest failure (cardiomegaly, pulmonary edema, jugular venous distention, hepatomegaly) as well as severe sequestration (in this patient), partial exchange transfusion is the preferred therapy. A target of 35 mL/kg of packed RBCs with a mean hematocrit of 70% to 75% can be expected to decrease the amount of sickling hemoglobin to 40% or less and to raise the hematocrit 15 points.

The patient in this case study had a normal chest x-ray.

The technique of partial exchange in this 5-year-old child would be to phlebotomize from one antecubital vein in increments of 50 mL, while concurrently 50 mL aliquots of donor blood is infused in the other antecubital vein. The blood should be warmed to at least room temperature and should be as fresh as possible. Exchange is continued until the 35 mL/kg limit of transfused blood is given. The patient must be continually monitored for vital signs and cardiac arrhythmia. Since acid citrate dextrose blood chelates calcium, baseline and serial calcium values should be obtained. During transfusion 5% dextrose should not be administered since acid citrate dextrose bank blood is rich in glucose. Following exchange, however, there is a risk of reactive hypoglycemia from the insulin stimulation of the exchange, so 10% dextrose is used as the IV solution and Dextrostix® is performed. Oxygen should be administered continuously. ABGs and electrolytes should be monitored.

The repletion of the volume deficit and the amelioration of the anemia usually reverse the sequestration process, with reduction of spleen size, alleviation of abdominal symptoms, and stabilization of vital signs and hematologic parameters.

This patient was admitted to the pediatric ICU for the completion of her exchange, as well as continuation of her antibiotic therapy. Her values after exchange transfusion were a hemoglobin of 8 g/dL, with a reticulocyte count of 17%. The heart stayed small, and there was no evidence on examination of congestive heart failure. Blood pressure, pulse, and respiratory rate all stabilized. A lumbar puncture was done in the ICU, which showed normal indices. All cultures were negative by the third day, and antibiotic therapy was discontinued.

Social services were consulted toward counseling and reeducation of this family regarding ongoing medical care.

The patient was discharged on the seventh hospital day, to be followed in a hematology clinic.

SUGGESTED READINGS

Bertram HL, Mentzer WC: Sickle cell disease. In Rudolph AM (ed): *Pediatrics,* ed 17. Norwalk, CT, Appleton-Century-Crofts, 1982, p 1068.

Lanzkowsky P: Sickle cell anemia. *Pediatr Clin North Am* 1979;26:925.

Lanzkowsky P, Shende A, Karaylein G, et al: Partial exchange transfusion in sickle cell anemia: Use in serious complications. *Am J Dis Child* 1978;132:1206.

Case 38

Six-year-old Female with Abdominal Pain

CASE PRESENTATION

A 6-year-old black female was well until she developed abdominal pain 18 hours before coming to the emergency department. The child awoke complaining of periumbilical pain at about 4 AM. The mother thought the child had eaten something bad and gave the child some Pepto-Bismol®, which was vomited about 15 minutes later. Because the child felt a little better she was put back to bed. The child awoke again at 7 AM with pain and shortly thereafter passed a small, loose stool. She vomited greenish material again at 8 AM. The child continued to have mild abdominal pain all day and stayed in bed, refusing all oral intake. The child began to cry about 8 PM, which prompted the mother to bring her to the emergency department. The child last urinated at 10 AM.

The prior medical history revealed the child had no major illnesses or hospitalizations in the past. Her immunizations were up to date.

Vital Signs

HR: 125 beats/min
RR: 20/min
BP: 100/65 mm Hg
T: 38.6°C (101.4°F)
WT: 21 kg

Physical Examination

GEN: Child refused to speak or smile while lying on the examination table with her knees drawn up

HEENT: *Eyes:* somewhat sunken; PERRLA; EOM intact; clear sclera; normal fundi. *Ears:* normal tympanic membranes. *Nose:* clear. *Oropharynx:* dry mouth; normal tonsils

NECK: Supple; shotty nodes

CHEST: Clear to percussion and auscultation; refusal to take deep breaths

CVS: Regular rhythm; grade II/VI systolic murmur loudest just below the right clavicle, which disappeared when the child was lying down

ABD: Bowel sounds heard only occasionally; no organomegaly or masses; tender to palpation over the entire abdomen; tapping on the abdominal wall caused child to scream; rebound only equivocally present; no costovertebral angle tenderness

GU: *Genitalia:* normal Tanner I, prepubertal female; no discharge noted. *Rectum:* nontender; no masses; small amount of soft stool; heme −

NEURO: Alert; oriented; normoreflexive; normal sensory, cranial nerve, and cerebellar examination

SKIN: Clear, but poor turgor

SUGGESTED INTERVENTIONS

1. Administer oxygen, 3 L/min, via nasal prongs.
2. Place IV with lactated Ringer's or normal saline 20 mL/kg; run in to reexpand the child's blood volume.
3. Order blood specimens for CBC, differential, sickle prep, amylase, electrolytes, creatinine, BUN, glucose, type and hold, blood culture, and Dextrostix® (result is 80 to 120 mg/dL).
4. Order urinalysis with urine saved for culture. Order stool culture.
5. Keep patient NPO.
6. Order abdominal series: upright chest, upright abdomen, and kidney/ureter/bladder (KUB) views.
7. Request surgical consultation.
8. Admit the patient.

CASE DISCUSSION

This child presented with abdominal pain and a history and physical examination compatible with 7% to 10% dehydration. After initial correction of the hypovolemia with 20 mL/kg of an isotonic fluid, the workup of her pain proceeded.

Vomiting and abdominal pain result from intra-abdominal processes as well as many extra-abdominal diseases. Sinusitis, pharyngitis, asthma, and pneumonia may all present as primarily abdominal symptoms. A complete physical examination and a chest x-ray will rule out these possibilities. Otitis media in infants also may result in vomiting and/or diarrhea.

Diabetes ketoacidosis also frequently presents with prominent vomiting and associated abdominal pain. No acetone was smelled on her breath, and the initial Dextrostix® test was normal. The results of her urinalysis proved negative for glucose and acetone.

Any disorder of the abdominal organs may be the source of the abdominal pain. Jaundice usually accompanies hepatitis, but a child may be anicteric. Liver function tests, prothrombin time, and a blood clot held for other serologies, such as a hepatitis panel and Epstein-Barr virus studies, generally comprise the evaluation of this entity. Pancreatitis is rare in children and usually causes symptoms for 3 or more weeks before diagnosis. Vomiting is prominent. Drugs, trauma, and familial hyperlipidemia are causes of abdominal pain in childhood.

Inflammatory bowel disease is usually indolent with symptoms and weight loss present for weeks to months before diagnosis. However, ulcerative colitis and Crohn's disease can present for the first time with sudden onset of toxic megacolon, which usually results in fever, tachycardia shock, abdominal pain, and distention. X-ray views of the abdomen show the colon dilated to more than 6 cm.

Various infections of the gut (particularly bacterial infections) can cause pain and vomiting. Diarrhea is usually prominent, but pain can precede diarrhea by as much as 18 to 24 hours. *Yersinia* is associated with the hyperplastic lymph nodes seen in mesenteric adenitis. *Campylobacter* causes particularly severe pain as well as bloody stools.

Familial Mediterranean fever, a recurrent inflammation of serosal surfaces, affects Armenians, Jews, and Arabs. The vast majority of patients have their first attack before age 20. Henoch-Schönlein purpura also causes abdominal pain, but the presence of characteristic dependent purpuric rash usually makes the diagnosis.

Female children *do* have ovaries, a fact that is sometimes overlooked. Torsion of the ovary and ovarian hernias are found in a significant number of young girls taken to surgery for a suspected appendicitis. In fact, 10% of children going to surgery for suspected appendicitis will have other serious surgical pathology causing their pain. Along with ovarian problems, perforation of Meckel's diverticulum, gallbladder disease, intussusception, and perforation due to severe bacterial infection account for most of the serious surgical pathologies.

Appendicitis is the most common cause of the surgical abdomen in school-age and adolescent children. However, infants occasionally develop appendicitis. These children appear septic and should be treated for sepsis. The presence of induration or discoloration of the right lower abdominal wall suggests appendicitis in an infant. Thickening of the wall may be seen on the x-ray film.

Older children usually give a history of periumbilical pain that localizes over several hours to the right lower quadrant. The younger the child the less likely it is that the pain will localize. There may be an episode or two of vomiting. At first, recently eaten food is vomited, then just gastric or bilious material. A small, loose stool may be passed, especially if the appendix is irritating the sigmoid colon.

The child walks bent over and lies quietly, often with legs partially flexed at the hip. Sudden movement such as jumping up and down or bumping the examination table intensifies the pain.

If the appendix ruptures, the child may experience transient relief of pain only to have recurrence of more severe and generalized abdominal pain. We noted a number of occasions when the presence of appendicitis was missed during this symptomatic interval. In general, diseases affecting the abdomen do not suddenly improve and a sudden disappearance of symptoms should be viewed as a warning sign.

The physical examination initially reveals a low-grade fever and perhaps mild tachycardia due to pain. If dehydration develops, signs of hypovolemia ensue. If frank shock is present due to appendiceal rupture, either from hypovolemic shock from third spacing in the inflamed peritoneum or distributive shock from sepsis, there will be marked tachycardia and hypotension, plus eventual changes in the sensorium.

The examination of the abdomen initially reveals diminished bowel sounds, which become absent if peritonitis develops. There may be generalized or local tenderness. It is helpful to palpate simultaneously both the right and left side using both hands. This allows subtle differences in guarding to be appreciated. Rebound is a late finding and indicates irritation of the parietal peritoneum. We find palpation of a child's abdomen sometimes facilitated by pressing the child's hand into his own abdominal wall. This gives them a sense of control, gives the physician some idea of what the abdomen feels like, and then has prepared the child for the physician's own examination. Maneuvers of the hips can be used, such as extension or flexion and abduction, which stretch the retroperitoneal muscles. The classic iliopsoas and obturator signs take advantage of this principle: the former indicative of processes lying on the psoas muscle, such as a retrocecal appendix, a psoas abscess, or perhaps a perinephric abscess, and the latter indicative of pelvic inflammatory processes, such as a pelvic appendix or a pelvic abscess.

A rectal examination is routinely performed, both to evaluate pelvic tenderness or mass and to determine if blood is present in the stool. Blood in the stool points toward infection, inflammatory bowel disease, intussusception, Meckel's diverticulum, or another nonappendiceal process. Some examiners prefer to defer the rectal examination until after the x-ray films are obtained. This prevents external air from being introduced into the rectum by the examining finger.

Laboratory determinations in acute appendicitis include a WBC count, which may show either a modest elevation of 10,000 to 12,000/cu mm or a shift toward immature forms. We routinely order that the amylase value be checked to rule out pancreatitis and that electrolytes, glucose, BUN, and creatinine determinations be performed to assess hydration and renal function. In cases of shock, a type and cross-match and ABGs should also be obtained. A urinalysis may show a few WBCs due to irritation of the ureter by the inflamed appendix, but there will be few to no bacteria. Very young infants may have major abnormalities of the urine, such as casts or proteinuria. These findings are consistent with any septic process and should not divert the examiner's attention away from the appendix. An upright film of the chest and abdomen is done to assess the possibility of perforation and obstruction. The plain supine film may show a fecalith in 5% to 10% of cases plus a scoliosis away from the appendix or blurring of the psoas shadow. If an abscess forms, it may create a mass effect and push the bowel aside.

An upright chest x-ray is taken to rule out pneumonia and air under the diaphragm from perforation.

The child should be kept NPO, and an IV for hydration should be begun. If vomiting is present, an NG tube should be inserted to empty the stomach. Any suspicion of perforation or obstruction demands insertion of an NG tube for proximal decompression.

Occasionally, the child will arrive with severe generalized peritonitis and in septic shock. Immediate resuscitation includes repeated boluses of Ringer's lactate and plasma expanders to correct hypotension, plus clindamycin, 25 to 40 mg/kg/day, IV, in divided doses every 6 hours; cefuroxime, 100 mg/kg/day, IV, in divided doses every 6 hours; and methylprednisolone, 2 mg/kg, IV, to treat the sepsis. Blood cultures are taken immediately prior to initiation of antibiotic therapy. Adequate blood must be cross-matched for the patient, and, as in severe trauma, we use a guideline of 100% total blood volume, which is approximately 8% of total body weight, or 80 mL/kg.

SUGGESTED READINGS

Knight PJ, Vassy LE: Specific diseases mimicking appendicitis in childhood. *Arch Surg* 1980;116:744.

Roy CC, Morin CL, Weber AM: Gastrointestinal emergency problems in paediatric practice. *Clin Gastroenterol* 1981;10:225.

Shaul WL: Clues to the early diagnosis of neonatal appendicitis. *J Pediatr* 1981;98:473.

Case 39

Six-year-old Female with Multiple Trauma

CASE PRESENTATION

A 6-year-old female was brought to the emergency department by the parents after having sustained blunt trauma to the abdomen inflicted by an automobile bumper. She had been struck after she ran between parked cars. The car was traveling approximately 25 mph. She was thrown to the ground on her left iliac region. There was no loss of consciousness, and she remembers the entire trip to the hospital. She was observed to ''lose her wind'' for several moments and now complains of a bad stomachache.

The child's past medical history was unremarkable. All her immunizations were up to date. She had no allergies, was not on any medications, and was never hospitalized for an illness or accident.

Vital Signs

BP: 90/70 mm Hg
P: 110 beats/min
RR: 38/min
WT: 22 kg (estimated)
T: 37°C (98.6°F)

Physical Examination

HEENT: *Head:* no evidence of basilar skull fracture; no obvious facial fracture; mandible and maxilla intact, with good occlusion. *Eyes:* EOM intact; sharp discs; no raccoon's eyes. *Ears:* no Battle's sign or hemotympanum. *Oropharynx:* moist mucous membranes

NECK: Supple; full range of motion through voluntary extension, flexion, lateral flexion, and rotation; no palpable tenderness or crepitance; midline trachea; no neck vein distention; no stridorous air passage

CHEST: Lungs clear; thorax nontender to anteroposterior and transverse compression; no crepitance; no palpable rib tenderness; intact sternum

CVS: Normal cardiac sounds; no gallop rhythm, rub, or crunch

ABD: Scaphoid, with no palpable hepatosplenomegaly; negative Trendelenburg sign; negative bowel sounds; no flank hematoma; no bruits heard over the anterior or posterior abdomen; negative Cullen's sign; no voluntary guarding; no rebound

GU: Good sphincter tone; brown stool; heme −; tenderness elicited to the left; ? positive left iliopsoas and obturator signs; palpation of the pelvis in lateral compression caused wincing

EXT: Palpation reveals no fractures, bruises, or dislocations; large abrasion with laceration on the lateral aspect of left thigh; resisted motion of the left leg, although no bony injury detected

SPINE: Entire thoracolumbosacral spine negative to palpation

NEURO: Alert, well-oriented female in moderate distress; motor, sensory, cranial nerve, cerebellum, and reflex examination normal

Vitals Signs After Physical Examination

BP: 70 mm Hg (systolic)
P: 128 beats/min

SUGGESTED INTERVENTIONS

1. Administer oxygen, 5 L/min, via nasal prongs.
2. Place two large-line angiocaths (no smaller than No. 18, No. 16 preferable) peripherally (antecubitals), hooked to lactated Ringer's through adult drippers, and run in rapidly until blood pressure normalizes to systolic of 95 mm Hg.
3. Place patient in Trendelenburg position with MAST suit placed under her ready to blow up.
4. Place indwelling Foley catheter; start measuring minute to minute urine output; order stat dipstick urine for heme, and send to laboratory for complete urinalysis.
5. Obtain blood specimens for type and cross-match six units, CBC, coagulogram, amylase, and ABGs.
6. Request stat surgical consultation.

7. Place NG tube; hook to continuous low suction; Gastroccult® first aspirant.
8. Perform pelvic and chest x-rays in trauma suite.

CASE DISCUSSION

A fractured pelvis is a frequently missed fracture, in general, but specifically in children. It is a major cause of post-traumatic mortality in children, and its associated retroperitoneal hematoma and bladder rupture are causes of unexplained shock, anemia, and infection. A high index of suspicion must always be kept in mind, especially for cases that are not as overt as this one.

The initial vital signs were suggestive. There was normal blood pressure but an unexplained tachycardia and a reduced pulse pressure. The respiratory rate was elevated, and in the absence of direct chest trauma, this must always be considered compensation for hypovolemia or hemorrhage until proven otherwise. Some centers recommend an ABG analysis, initially to look for the early base deficit associated with hemorrhage.

Obtaining postural vital signs would have been a good idea at this point to elicit the occult hypotension. The tilt test is a good indicator of traumatic hemorrhagic shock. A prudent physician would have had lines started and blood samples sent at this point of the evaluation, before the entire examination was completed. The use of Ringer's lactate as the initial resuscitation medium cannot be emphasized too strongly. Children need rapid flow rates when their blood pressures suddenly decompensate, so use adult tubing and drip chambers in trauma.

The craniocervical examination was noncontributory. The cardiothoracic examination was also suggestive of impending hypovolemic shock, in that the respiratory rate was up and the lungs were perfectly clear. Also, the finding of an increased cardiac first sound (S_1) should always suggest decreased intravascular volume.

The abdominal examination appeared normal and really did not suggest splenic or hepatic injury. The findings of scaphoid abdomen, absence of guarding, but presence of bowel sounds all mitigated against intestinal perforation and intraperitoneal blood, bile, or feces. The negative Trendelenburg test (placing the patient in Trendelenburg position and looking for shoulder radiation of pain) was against free intraperitoneal blood, bile, or intestinal contents.

The rectal examination (mandatory in trauma) was the first indication of a pathologic problem, and the finding of tenderness along the left side should intensify the suspicion of a fractured pelvis. The absence of a concomitant mass does not rule out pelvic or retroperitoneal hematoma. In males the prostate must be specifically felt and defined, since traumatic rupture of the prostatic urethra is associated with a ''missing'' prostate and a boggy tender mass in its place.

A thorough examination of the pelvis always includes palpation of the entire bony structure and compression in both anteroposterior and transverse directions to elicit tenderness and/or instability. The sacroiliac joints should be examined.

Pelvic bimanual examination in sexually active females should always be done to uncover trauma to the internal genitalia, as well as to pick up physical findings of coexisting pregnancy. Urine and serum pregnancy tests should accompany other studies in such female patients.

The absence of bony tenderness on direct palpation fairly well ruled out extremity fracture/dislocation, but the pain on motion of the left leg must be explained. Femoral shaft or head acetabular, pelvic ring, sacroiliac, and lumbosacral injuries would all be possible with this finding. A retroperitoneal/pelvic hematoma on the left alone could have caused this sign.

The results of neurologic examination were apparently within normal limits, but even an initially normal distal motor, sensory, and reflex examination does not rule out pelvic nerve injury.

The urinalysis in this case showed 30 to 50 RBCs per high-powered field; there were no other abnormalities in the urine. The initial hematocrit on admission was 39% but fell to 28% within 1 hour. The amylase value and coagulogram were normal.

An initial chest x-ray done semiupright in the trauma suite revealed a small heart and very clear lungs, but the stat anteroposterior pelvic x-ray revealed left inferior and superior pubic rami fracture as well as a question of a widening left sacroiliac joint. The surgeon in consultation recommended external stabilization of the pelvis using a Harrison fixation device, abdominal CT, and pelvic angiographic study in the radiology suite following hemodynamic stabilization. The patient was transfused with 3 units of whole blood in the emergency department, and her hematocrit stabilized at 32%. Her blood pressure normalized (with negative tilt test), and she was taken for CT angiography, during which a large left pelvic hematoma and bleeding arteries were identified. All other abdominal viscera were normal. Bleeding vessels were embolized with Silastic® spherules under direct angiographic visualization.

Following the angiography, a cystogram was done through the Foley catheter using 15 mL/kg of Conray-30®. This revealed extrinsic compression from the pelvic hematoma and showed no ruptured bladder. All pertinent views were obtained to rule out even the slightest extravasation of contrast medium. The abdominal CT with contrast had revealed no renal/ureteral injury, and it had been elected not to select the renal arteries for further angiographic study. The urologic diagnosis became bladder contusion.

The patient had a very stable postangiographic course and was taken to the PICU.

A fractured pelvis is seen frequently in pediatric blunt trauma. The usual inciting events are motor vehicle accidents, with the child usually being the pedestrian; in falls from a height, usually in excess of 10 feet; and in straddle injuries. Associated injuries are common and include bladder injury, urethral injury, rectal laceration, and pelvic hematoma. Major vessel injury is seen in approximately 3% of cases. Of interest is the fact that there is a 25% incidence of head injury in cases of pelvic fracture, and this underlies the type of mechanism of injury forceful enough to fracture the pelvis.

The most frequently fractured pelvic bones in children are the pubic rami (as in this case), the acetabulum, diastasis of the sacroiliac joints, and ischial tuberosity fractures.

Forty percent of pediatric patients need transfusions, with the average amount being 6 units. The overall mortality approximates 5%, with hemorrhage and delayed infection being the usual causes.

Therapy is always directed at stabilization of the pelvis. The pediatric MAST suit has been used quite successfully in unstable cases with large hemorrhages. Other surgical procedures directed at opening the hematoma directly and ligating the bleeding vessels have fallen into disrepute. Newer techniques of angiographic embolization and obliteration are showing very promising results. Occasionally the hypogastric vessels are ligated for massive hemorrhage.

SUGGESTED READINGS

Clark SS, Prudencio RF: Lower urinary tract injuries associated with pelvic fractures. *Surg Clin North Am* 1972;52:183.

Cowley MD, Dunham CM: Pelvic fractures. In Maryland Institute for Emergency Medical Services: *Shock and Trauma Manual.* Baltimore, University Park Press, 1982, pp 193–199.

Dunn EL, Berry PH, Connally JD: Computed tomography of the pelvis in trauma. *J Trauma* 1983;23:3787.

Garcia V, Eichelberger MR, Ziegler M, et al: Use of MAST suit in child with fractured pelvis. *J Pediatr Surg* 1981;16:544.

Haller JA, Reichard SA, Shorter, N, et al: Pelvic fractures in children: Review of 120 cases. *J Pediatr Surg* 1980;15:727.

Trunkey DD, Chapman MW, Lim RC, et al: Management of pelvic fractures in blunt trauma. *J Trauma* 1974;14:912.

Case 40

Six-year-old Male with Scrotal Pain

CASE PRESENTATION

A 6-year-old male was playing with friends when he jumped off a small hillside, landed on his feet, and felt an acute pain in his left scrotum. He was brought to the emergency department 1 hour later by his mother who stated that the child has a very tender scrotal sac.

Vital Signs

BP: 90/56 mm Hg
HR: 95 beats/min
RR: 17/min
T: 38°C (100.4°F)
WT: 22 kg

Physical Examination

GEN: Well-developed, well-nourished alert male in mild discomfort.
HEENT: *Head:* normocephalic. *Eyes:* PERRLA; EOM intact; normal discs. *Ears:* normal tympanic membranes. *Nose:* without drainage. *Throat:* pink, no exudate
NECK: Supple with pea-sized cervical adenopathy bilaterally
CHEST: Lungs symmetrically clear
CVS: Regular rhythm: no rub, murmur, or gallop rhythm

ABD: Soft; no masses; normal bowel sounds; +/− diffuse abdominal
        tenderness, slightly increased in the right lower quadrant; no
        rebound; no costovertebral angle tenderness
GU: Scrotal sac erythematous, +/− edema on the left; unable to appreci-
        ate mass; moderate to severe pain on palpation; unable to appreciate
        detail of left testis secondary to tenderness and swelling; negative
        transillumination; no relief of pain on elevation of testis. Right testis
        normal
EXT: Full range of motion; no cyanosis; no clubbing; no edema
NEURO: Grossly intact
SKIN: No rash or petechiae

SUGGESTED INTERVENTIONS

1. Order CBC with differential; perform urinalysis.
2. Keep patient NPO.
3. Start IV with 5% dextrose in 0.25 normal saline at maintenance rate of
   65 mL/hr
4. Attempt manual detorsion, after analgesic, such as morphine sulfate,
   0.1 mg/kg, IV, with naloxone (Narcan®) on standby (0.01 to 0.02 mg/kg,
   IV).
5. Request immediate consultation with urologist or pediatric surgeon.

CASE DISCUSSION

An acute painful swelling of the scrotum in childhood is a medical emergency.
The differential diagnosis needs to be considered without delay and therapy
initiated to prevent testicular loss.

Torsion of the intrascrotal relics of the mesonephric and paramesonephric ducts
most commonly affects the appendix and epididymis. These two appendices can
either be sessile or pedunculated. If pedunculated, the appendix can twist around
its base, leading to venous engorgement, swelling, and infarction.

As in true testicular torsion, the onset of pain is sudden. If the child is seen early
after the onset of pain, one may be able to feel a small tender lump at the
superolateral pole of the testicle or epididymis with no testicular or epididymal
enlargement or pain.

The classic "blue dot" sign of infarcted appendage may be seen by stretching
the scrotal skin over the lump. However, this sign is unreliable secondary to
scrotal edema.

If a confident diagnosis of testicular appendage torsion can be made, surgery is
not indicated since the infarcted appendix rapidly atrophies and the symptoms

subside without sequelae. These children should receive analgesics and bed rest and return in 24 to 48 hours for a repeat examination.

Torsion of the spermatic chord has two peak periods of occurrence: during the perinatal period and the other around puberty. Three anatomic types are recognized when the testis is fully descended:

1. Supravaginal torsion: the chord twists above the tunica vaginalis with strangulation of the serous sac. This condition is seen in newborns, at which time the tunica vaginalis has only loose attachments to the scrotal wall.
2. Intravaginal torsion: this is the most common form of torsion and is caused by a congenital deformity of the tunica vaginalis. The tunica covers the entire epididymis and extends high on the spermatic chord so there is inadequate fixation of the testis and epididymis to the intrascrotal tissue. This is the description of the classic "bell clapper" deformity.
3. Torsion of the mesorchium between the testis and epididymis: this a rare cause of torsion and occurs when the testis and epididymis are widely separated.

The etiology of torsion is unknown. A strong contraction of the spirally arranged cremasteric fibers has been suggested; however, frequently torsion occurs while the child is asleep. The symptoms are usually sudden, and pain may be experienced first in the central abdomen, iliac fossa, or groin with associated nausea and vomiting. This presentation is often confused with abdominal pathology. There may exist a history of similar mild attacks of "abdominal pain" that resolved spontaneously. On examination the testis is swollen, firm, and extremely tender. The affected testis may be lying higher than its contralateral mate. This sign is inconsistent because the abnormal local anatomy that predisposes to intravaginal torsion may exist in fact bilaterally.

The safe interval of time between the onset of symptoms in torsion of the testis and irreversible testicular damage is unknown. In experimental testicular ischemia a progressive loss of germinal and Sertoli cells is seen within 4 to 6 hours, with death of Leydig cells after 10 hours. All investigators seem to agree that testicular salvage is a time-related phenomenon and advocate an aggressive approach to diagnosis and treatment.

Newer techniques of assessment of torsion have been developed over the past decade. These include Doppler flow studies, scrotal perfusion isotopic scanning, and fluorescein staining.

Millaret and Liaras, in 1974, first applied the Doppler principle to the differential diagnosis of the acute scrotum. The Doppler instrument emits a constant beam of ultrasonic waves that is directed at moving cells and fluid within blood vessels. An increase, decrease, or absence of blood flow in the testis can readily be detected.

In the patient with symptoms of 4 to 12 hours in duration a quick decision about vascular status may be reached with the aid of the Doppler flow studies and decisions about viability made.

Scrotal imaging with technetium Tc 99m is useful in the diagnosis of torsion of the testicle based on the knowledge that in torsion the testicle has impaired blood supply and therefore decreased perfusion. Increased uptake should be recorded in areas of increased perfusion resulting from inflammation exemplified in the scrotum by epididymitis. Isotope scans are best interpreted by comparing the angiographic phase and the delayed tissue phase; thereby not only is an image recorded, but function and relative vascularity can be estimated. However, small testicles in small children can limit the diagnostic capabilities of the scan. Areas of decreased isotope uptake may represent a nonperfused testicle compatible with torsion, a hematoma in the scrotal wall or testicular capsule, an abscess, a hydrocele, or a necrotic tumor. Increased activity is found in mostly inflammatory conditions such as epididymo-orchitis both in the dynamic portion of the scan and in the static delayed images. Torsion of the testicular appendages may produce slightly increased perfusion, but the scrotal structures frequently appear normal. Scrotal scanning does not replace a complete evaluation from an experienced urologist or pediatric surgeon. It must be stressed, however, that many urologists will not risk the time necessary to organize, accomplish, and evaluate testicular scans. Many advocate an ''operate on suspicion'' policy.

Fluorescent staining is utilized as an intraoperative aid in testicular salvage after detorsion. Fluorescence of the testis or tunica albuginea within 5 to 10 minutes after IV injection correlates well with testicular viability following detorsion as detected by Wood's light.

If a child is seen within 1 to 2 hours after the onset of torsion, and has minimal scrotal swelling, manual detorsion of the spermatic cord may be performed. Morphine sulfate, 0.1 mg/kg, IV, administered prior to the procedure will allow for better cooperation. A majority of torsion occurs in a medial direction, so detorsion should be attempted with rotation outward to the thigh. Manual reduction may relieve the surgical emergency but does not eliminate the need for urologic or pediatric surgical intervention for permanent fixation.

Acute epididymitis is uncommon in prepubertal males. In a young child it may complicate a urinary tract infection, but usually only when there preexists anatomical abnormalities that allow infection to spread along the vas deferens. The enlarged epididymis may be palpable as swelling distinct from the testis, initially, but as the infection spreads, the inflammation of the testis and scrotal sac prevents accurate diagnosis. Elevation of the scrotum is said to relieve the pain in epididymo-orchitis (Prehn's sign), but this sign is very unreliable in children and does not aid in the differentiation of the scrotal swelling from torsions. The presence of pyuria and bacteriuria should help clarify the diagnosis but are not consistently present. Treatment with the appropriate antibiotic (e.g., trimethoprim-sulfamethoxarole) will achieve good epididymal tissue penetration. Prevention of recurrence requires the correction of the underlying urologic abnormality.

Idiopathic scrotal edema is a rare clinical entity seen in males between 5 and 10 years of age. The edema spreads rapidly, involving one or, less often, both sides of the scrotum. The affected hemiscrotum becomes firm and bright pink. Often the swelling and discoloration extend to the groin, perineum, and/or penis. There is local erythema but little pain. The appearance is that of a low-grade cellulitis, but there is no fever, the total WBC count is normal, and the edema fluid is sterile on culture. An allergic phenomenon has been hypothesized and occasionally supported by peripheral eosinophilia. The edema resolves quickly over 48 hours without treatment and is known to recur.

A petechial rash and scrotal edema are often the presenting signs of Henoch-Schönlein purpura, a nonthrombocytopenic purpura. The rash usually is first noted on the lower extremities and buttocks. The scrotal contents are usually not involved, but swelling can be severe enough to obscure diagnosis.

Any painless, firm scrotal swelling is suspicious of tumor. Under 2 years of age, the primary tumor of concern is yolk-sac carcinoma; after puberty, a germinal cell tumor should be considered.

SUGGESTED READINGS

Allan WR: The testis-torsion and trauma. *Practitioner* 1982;226:1837.

Hemalatha V, Ricxkwood AMK: The diagnosis and management of acute scrotal conditions in boys. *Br Med J* 1981;53:455.

Millaret R, Liaras H: Ultrasonic diagnosis and therapy of torsion of the testis. *J Chir* 1974;107:35.

Ransler CW, Allen TD: Torsion of the spermatic chord. *Urol Clin North Am* 1982;9:245.

Smith SP, King LR: Torsion of the testis: Techniques of assessment. *Urol Clin North Am* 1979;6:429.

Case 41

Six-year-old Male with Rash, Arthralgia, and Scrotal Pain

CASE PRESENTATION

A 6-year-old male presented at 4 PM in the emergency department because a sudden onset of severe testicular pain on the left began 1 hour before arrival. There was no history of trauma to the perineal area and no previous operations or known abnormalities. The child was normal until 2 days previously when he complained of pain in his knees, which resolved over the next day. His parents did not recall any swelling or redness of the joints. Yesterday the child complained of abdominal pain several times off and on. He slept poorly because of the pain, but this problem had not been present for the past 8 to 10 hours. The child also refused to walk since the morning because "it hurt." No specific area of pain causing this had been elicited.

The parents stated the child had not been sick recently and was taking no medications. There was no fever, vomiting, or diarrhea.

The past medical history was noncontributory, and his immunizations were up to date.

Vital Signs

T: 36.9°C (98.4°F)
HR: 95 beats/min
RR: 18/min
BP: 100/65 mm Hg
WT: 21 kg

Physical Examination

GEN: Alert, but mildly distressed child
HEENT: Normal examination

233

NECK: Supple with shotty adenopathy

CHEST: Clear to percussion and auscultation

CVS: Regular; no murmur or S_1 and S_2

ABD: Not tender; normal bowel sounds; no masses or organomegaly

GU: *Genitalia:* normal circumcised male penis; ecchymosis present in skin of left side of scrotum; testis on left was tender to palpation. *Rectum:* normal tone; stool heme −

EXT: No swelling of joints; pain to motion of right knee and both ankles

NEURO: Intact cranial nerves II through XI; peripheral strength intact; refusal to walk; deep tendon reflexes +2 and symmetric; downgoing toes

SKIN: Several small purpuric palpable lesions scattered on ankles and feet ranging from a few millimeters to 0.5 cm

SUGGESTED INTERVENTIONS

1. Order blood specimens for CBC, differential, platelet count, ESR, prothrombin time, partial thromboplastin time, BUN, creatinine, C3 complement level, streptozyme.
2. Perform urinalysis; hold sample for possible culture.
3. Order abdominal series: upright chest and abdomen films.
4. Request urology and general surgery consultations.
5. Admit the patient.

CASE DISCUSSION

Henoch-Schönlein purpura is a vasculitic syndrome that typically affects children from infancy through early adolescence. Rare cases have been described in adults. The disorder may occasionally follow a variety of infections or environmental agents, including *Streptococcus, Mycoplasma, Yersinia,* hepatitis B, foods, drugs, insect bites, and cold exposure. Despite this long list, the etiology for a specific case is seldom determined.

The typical rash may be preceded for 1 or 2 days by a maculopapular or urticarial rash. The rash of Henoch-Schönlein purpura is a tender, generally dependent, palpable purpura generally found on the buttocks and legs. However, the rash may involve any skin surface especially in younger children. Nonspecific swelling of subcutaneous tissue may also occur. Arthralgia accompanies the rash 70% to 80% of the time and may precede its onset by as long as 2 weeks. Although very painful the arthralgia is self-limited and leaves no residual damage. Bed rest and analgesia are sufficient.

The incidence of orchitis associated with Henoch-Schönlein purpura is reported to be between 38% and 1%. This wide range most likely reflects the amount of selection bias based on a referral versus a primary care practice. In the presence of testicular pain, especially with ecchymotic lesion, the physician should ask diligently about other symptoms associated with Henoch-Schönlein purpura. The orchitis of Henoch-Schönlein purpura is associated with subsequent testicular torsion, so when actual testicular involvement is present clinically a urologist should be consulted to rule out possible torsion.

The GI system also becomes involved in 50% of cases with pain and occult bleeding. Five percent of these patients will develop an intussusception due to a hematoma acting as a leading point. Perforations of the gut wall may be a very rare event.

This child had negative abdominal x-rays and was cleared by the general surgeon.

Gross or microscopic hematuria develops in 40% of patients and may or may not be associated with nonspecific proteinuria. Microscopic hematuria by itself is usually benign while patients with gross hematuria or proteinuria plus hematuria (gross or microscopic) have a 10% to 20% risk of long-term renal abnormalities. Once nephritis and the nephrotic syndrome are established the child has a 50% risk of developing chronic renal insufficiency. Patients with gross hematuria also seem to have more recurrences of their rash. If the rash does recur, the symptoms are similar to the original rash but shorter lived and milder.

This patient had no proteinuria, but 20 RBCs per high-powered field. The BUN and creatinine values were normal.

Elevated levels of serum IgA are found in 50% of patients, but this finding is not helpful prognostically. In fact, there are no specific tests for Henoch-Schönlein purpura. Since coagulopathies, infectious diseases, neoplasms, and allergic reactions may mimic this disorder, laboratory work is needed to rule out these disorders. Occasional patients may need serum immunoglobins, ASO titers or streptozymes, antinuclear antibody, rheumatoid factors, and/or total hemolytic complement factor determinations.

Other rare complications of this disease include seizures or CNS bleeding, peripheral neuritis, orchitis, eye involvement, pulmonary hemorrhage, and carditis.

Most patients do well, with the rash disappearing while the child is at bed rest only to reappear when walking begins. This cycle may occur over several months before total resolution. Even after apparent total resolution there may be another recurrence up to 6 months later. The parents should be informed about abdominal pain and the possibility of intussusception. Definite pediatric follow-up for serial urinalysis is necessary to identify those children who progress to chronic nephritis. Corticosteroids (prednisone, 1 to 2 mg/kg/day) have been used to alleviate the abdominal and joint pain as well as severe hemorrhagic manifestations but they do not change the course of the purpuric rash or nephritis.

The diagnosis of Henoch-Schönlein purpura rests heavily on the presence of the characteristic rash, urinalysis, abdominal pain, and joint manifestations. Other causes of purpura such as septicemia (especially meningococcemia), hemolytic uremia syndrome, and coagulopathies should be considered. Collagen vascular disorders, especially systemic lupus erythematosus, may also present with a similar rash. However, appropriate serologic tests plus the presence of other characteristics of systemic lupus suggest the correct diagnosis.

This patient had an uneventful course and had amelioration of his hematuria in 1 week, without development of nephrotic syndrome, hypertension, or azotemia. All other GI and joint symptoms similarly disappeared. He was discharged to the care of his private medical doctor.

SUGGESTED READINGS

Harvey JG, Colditz PB: Henoch-Schönlein purpura: A surgical review. *Aust Paediatr J* 1984;20:13.

Loh HS, Jalan OM: Testicular torsion in Henoch-Schönlein syndrome. *Br Med J* 1974;2:96.

Martinez-Frontanilla LA: Surgical complications in Henoch-Schönlein purpura. *J Pediatr Surg* 1984;19:434.

O'Regan S, Robitaille P: Orchitis mimicking testicular torsion in Henoch-Schönlein purpura. *J Urol* 1981;126:834.

Saulsbury FT: Henoch-Schönlein purpura. *Pediatr Derm* 1984;1:195.

Case 42

Seven-year-old Male with Anisocoria and Obtundation

CASE PRESENTATION

A 7-year-old male fell from his skateboard onto a concrete pavement striking his right temple approximately 1 hour prior to presentation in the emergency department. He had definite transient loss of consciousness lasting approximately 3 minutes by witnessed observation. He gradually regained full consciousness but kept perseverating on certain phrases (e.g., "Where am I?").

He was initially noted to have a scalp hematoma over the right temple but was not complaining of any pain, motor, or sensory problem and went home without obtaining medical attention.

He came home promptly whereupon his mother noted the bruised temple. In the middle of his (confused) explanation, he lapsed once again into unconsciousness. The mother quickly called the paramedics.

On presentation in the emergency department the patient was obtunded, with an obviously dilated right pupil. He was breathing spontaneously. The paramedics had "scooped and hauled" the patient to the emergency department and no advanced life support was initiated.

Vital Signs

BP: 120/80 mm Hg
P: 55 beats/min
RR: 10/min
T: No tactile temperature
WT: 24 kg (estimated)

Physical Examination

GEN: Comatose male child appearing otherwise well developed and well nourished, breathing shallowly, with intermittently decorticate posturing on the left

HEENT: *Head:* large (5 × 5 cm) hematoma overlying right temporal squama; no depression noted; no bruit heard; no other scalp lesion noted; facial bones all intact. *Eyes:* left pupil 5 mm, mid position; right pupil 9 mm, nonreactive; normal fundi; Doll's eyes reflex deferred; negative corneal reflex; no raccoon's eyes. *Ears:* no Battle's sign; no hemotympanum, no discharge. *Nose:* no discharge. *Oropharynx:* tongue in midline; no gag reflex

NECK: No palpable bony deformity or crepitance; neck in axial traction; midline trachea; no neck vein distention; no stridor. Neck was "sandbagged" after examination

CHEST: Full excursion of chest wall with inspiration; no paradox; symmetric sounds; no bony lesions; no crepitance over ribs; no rales or rhonchi; tactile fremitus normal and symmetric; no sternal deformity; full diaphragmatic excursion; occasional apneusic episodes

CVR: Regular rhythm; cardiac rate of 60 beats/min; no murmur, gallop rhythm, or rub; point of maximal impulse normally located

ABD: Scaphoid; absent bowel sounds; no mass; no hepatosplenomegaly; no bruises; no gross deformity; no distraction on anteroposterior and lateral compression

GU: *Rectum:* normal tone; heme negative; prostate in normal location

EXT: All located without obvious deformity; no wound; no cyanosis; no edema

NEURO: Comatose; no response to verbal command; decorticate flexion response to noxious stimulus; Glasgow Coma Scale score of 5; tone increased in left upper and left lower extremities; left lower extremity in external rotated posture; Babinski sign asymmetric with dorsiflexion on left; four-beat clonus detected in left lower extremity

SUGGESTED INTERVENTIONS

1. Immediately stabilize airway, maintaining neck in sniffing position, with California collar applied, oropharyngeal airway inserted, and patient mask ventilated with 100% oxygen.
2. Place on cardiac monitor.
3. Start peripheral large IV line (No. 18 angiocath started in left antecubital vein) with normal saline at KVO.

4. Obtain blood specimens for type and cross-match 4 units whole blood, CBC, prothrombin time, partial thromboplastin time, baseline electrolytes, osmolarity, and glucose. Dextrostix® = 90 to 120 mg/dL.
5. After adequate preoxygenation (2 minutes), give pancuronium, 0.48 mg (0.02 mg/kg) IVp; atropine, 0.48 mg (0.02 mg/kg) IVp; thiopental, 96 mg (4 mg/kg) IVp; and lidocaine, 24 mg (1 mg/kg) IVp.
6. After pulse increases (showing atropinization effect), give succinylcholine, 48 mg (2 mg/kg) IVp. Apply pressure to the cricoid ring (the Selleck maneuver), and intubate the patient 1 minute later with a No. 6 uncuffed Portex tube. Hyperventilation is initiated as soon as tube position is confirmed by physical examination.
7. Start mannitol (20%) infusion, 240 mL (2 g/kg), IVFD over 10 minutes.
8. Order ABGs. Volume ventilation is adjusted to achieve P_{CO_2} in the range of 23 to 25 mm Hg.
9. Place a Foley catheter. Have initial urine sample dipped for heme; send for urinalysis; Urimeter® marked at time zero; monitor urine output continuously.
10. Additional medications: furosemide (Lasix®), 24 mg (1 mg/kg) IVp; dexamethasone (Decadron®), 10 mg IVp.
11. Order lateral cross-table cervical spine x-ray (must see down to C7 level).
12. Place NG tube. Order Gastroccult®. Hook to low continuous suction.
13. Order chest x-ray (portable, semi-upright).
14. Request stat neurosurgical consultation.
15. Admit the patient.

CASE DISCUSSION

This patient showed the classic signs, symptoms, and progression of serious intracranial bleeding—most likely acute epidural hematoma. The initial insult, followed by a short lucid interval, culminating in an irreversible progressive deterioration of mental function with a dilating unilateral pupil, is a textbook description of this lethal entity.

This patient's initial vital signs and coma confirmed Cushing's triad: hypertension, slow pulse, and deteriorated level of consciousness. The slow respiratory rate and apneusis are further evidence of increased cerebral pressure. The large temporal squamal hematoma ipsilateral to the dilating pupil and contralateral to the apparent long tract signs strongly suggests a right-sided epidural hematoma, with the right middle meningeal artery lacerated by a probable fracture throughout this weakened portion of the temporal bone. A herniating right uncus most likely accounts for the constellation of signs and symptoms found in this child. The correlation of dilating pupil and/or hemiparesis to the side of the epidural has frequently led the clinician astray and has been variably reported to be misleading in a significant number of cases. Also, epidural hematomas (acute) are seen bilaterally in approximately 40% of cases, and therefore the signs indicating "sidedness" really only indicate the lobe herniating first. A high index of suspicion must be held out for bilaterality, and no one can be certain about the location of the actual hematoma based on physical findings alone.

The initial resuscitation of this patient included placing him in the most ideal position for his cervical spine stability, as well as airway patency: this is the "sniffing" position, with neither neck extension or flexion but with the occiput anteriorly displaced approximately 2 inches. This is easily effected by placing a flat folded towel under the occiput. Towel rolls under the nape should be avoided because of their tendency to hyperextend the neck. Axial traction should be applied until a definitive collar or sandbags can be used to achieve stability. Semiflexible plastic collars such as the Philadelphia or California collars, or the more rigid four-poster collars, are very difficult to use in infants and small children, generally aged 5 and under. In this 7-year-old male a California collar should have presented no difficulty.

The essence of this resuscitation was airway management and cerebral resuscitation. The sequence of events for the placement of the endotracheal tube highlight some important points about the pediatric victim of head trauma.

Adequate initial oxygenation was maintained in the sniffing position with bag and mask ventilation using an oropharyngeal airway. The correct size of such an airway should equal the length from the corner of the child's mouth to the angle of that ipsilateral mandible. Next a peripheral angiocath was started in an antecubital location. This site is easy to enter and can ensure a fairly large catheter. We avoid butterfly catheters in our critically injured and ill children and recommend general adoption of this rule. Blood samples are sent for diagnostic study as well as typing and cross-matching (see Suggested Interventions No. 4). The best IV fluid for intracerebral injury is full-strength crystalloid run at KVO. This ensures that a minimum of free water is transferred to the injured brain, therefore forestalling edema formation. For true "KVO" flow, a pump must be used in the IV circuit and set to the minimum. Incidentally, in cases of multiple trauma, when there is head injury combined with serious other visceral injury and the patient is in hypovolemic hemorrhagic shock, full-strength crystalloid is still the resuscitation fluid of choice, opened up wide until blood pressure normalizes. For the emergency department physician who initially sees a child with an isolated head injury or one associated with multiple trauma, the IV fluid decision is easy: full-strength crystalloid (e.g., normal saline or lactated Ringer's).

We see no reason in this case to initiate resuscitation with a central venous pressure line, Swan-Ganz catheter, or arterial line. It is our belief that these lines can be done as a secondary (delayed) intervention and in this case are not indicated as primary resuscitation maneuvers.

It is very important that children with suspected increased cerebral pressure needing cerebral resuscitation and airway protection be paralyzed prior to intubation unless specific contraindication exists. Upper airway obstruction constitutes the major contraindication to paralysis. Children who struggle and actively fight intubation are known to rapidly raise their already elevated cerebral pressure, frequently with disastrous consequence. Prior paralysis blocks this effect. Obviously flaccid victims (Glasgow Coma Score = 3) do not need to be paralyzed. Ideal preparation for paralysis and intubation is to adequately preoxygenate with bag-mask ventilation using 100% FIo_2 and with an oropharyngeal airway in place. To effect paralysis, we use a drug sequence according to the mnemonic "PATS"—*P*ancuronium-*A*tropine-*T*hiopental-*S*uccinylcholine. Pancuronium is administered in a defasciculating dosage, not a paralyzing dosage, of 0.02 mg/kg. The main disadvantages of succinylcholine are related to its depolarizing action, which causes major muscular fasciculation. This precipitates increased intracranial pressure, hyperkalemia, acidosis, bone fractures, glaucoma, vomiting and aspiration, and occasional frank arrest. These all can be prevented by prior defasciculation with competitive agents such as pancuronium or curare at less than paralyzing dosages. Atropine is given next, as long as the patient's baseline pulse rate is not in excess of 200 beats/min. The dosage is 0.02 mg/kg IV (this is the same dosage as pancuronium), and we never give less than a minimum dose of 0.15 mg to avoid the low-dose paradox (parasympathomimesis) of atropine. Next, thiopental is given intravenously (4 mg/kg) to further ablate increased cerebral pressure and to induce some amnesis. This drug is strictly contraindicated if the patient is hypotensive, perhaps as a result of blood loss from other related trauma. We relatively contraindicate thiopental in multiple trauma, where barbiturate-induced hypotension could be confused with ongoing hemorrhagic shock and therapeutic interventions are delayed. After these premedications are given and the pulse rate shows an increase indicating atropine effect, we finally administer succinylcholine at a dose of 2 mg/kg IV while simultaneously pressing on the cricoid cartilage (Selleck maneuver) and maintaining oxygenation. One minute later, the child is intubated via the oropharyngeal approach route, with an assistant using axial traction (cephalad) on the cervical spine. This is a perfectly safe method of airway control, even with the suspicion of underlying spine injury. Children can be safely intubated in this manner without undue extension or flexion of the cervical spine. The severe complications of emergency cricothyroidotomy in children make this procedure undesirable unless absolutely necessary for airway control not amenable from above. With surgical expertise available, an emergency tracheostomy is always preferable to cricothyroidotomy in childhood.

Blind nasotracheal intubation is virtually impossible in younger children (generally age 7 and under).

Once the tube is placed, its position is confirmed by auscultation of both chests and stomach. Final confirmation must await the results of the chest film. This should always be done since smaller children can mask misplacement if breath sounds alone are relied on.

We favor hyperventilation to a Pco_2 of 23 to 25 mm Hg to minimize cerebral blood flow and consequent cerebral edema.

The next significant intervention is the infusion of 2 g/kg of mannitol given as 20% solution and infused over 10 to 15 minutes. Remember that a Foley catheter must be in place already or put in shortly after initiation of the infusion (see Suggested Intervention No. 9).

We believe strongly that, despite the debate over rebound hyperemia, and possible violation of the blood–brain barrier through trauma, that the immediate life-saving reduction in intracranial pressure that is accomplished by mannitol infusion may buy enough time to get the patient to surgery (with or without an intervening head CT scan), so that discussions of delayed rebound are not germane to the emergency department physician who must keep the patient alive through this acute herniation of the brain. Rebound may be safely managed in the ICU setting through a multitude of monitoring and therapeutic interventions. We also use furosemide, 1 mg/kg, as an auxiliary dehydrating agent. This also makes use of the Foley catheter mandatory, as well as ongoing knowledge of the fluid and electrolyte status of the patient (see Suggested Intervention No. 4).

The use of dexamethasone in acutely decompensating tentorial herniation syndromes is still controversial. However, it is used at our institution at a dose of approximately 0.5 mg/kg, usually not exceeding 10 mg.

The portable cervical spine x-ray is necessary in this patient, who did receive enough trauma to induce a probable epidural hematoma and who is currently comatose. It is important to realize that cervical cord trauma in general is a rather rare event in the pediatric population and that this patient manifested no cervical symptoms prior to the acute decompensation; nevertheless the onus is on the emergency department physician to exonerate injury to the cervical spine. Accordingly, all maneuvers and procedures done to this point were done with spinal precautions. The ABCs of this resuscitation were completed prior to any x-ray study. The lateral cervical spine film is done with one assistant pulling down on the arms, while a second assistant applies countertraction at the chin in a cephalad axial direction, keeping hands out of the direct x-ray pathway. This will usually guarantee a good spine x-ray, at least down to the C7 level. If this approach is not adequate, a portable swimmer's view is indicated. The NG tube is placed next, after the cervical spine film was read as negative. Finally, the portable, upright chest x-ray is taken to confirm endotracheal tube and NG tube placement, as well as to delineate any traumatic, iatrogenic, or preexisting thoracic problem.

This patient responded very well to the cerebral resuscitation protocol, reversing his dilated pupil and achieving a Glasgow Coma Score of approximately 10.

He was stable enough for CT scan of the head, which led to a diagnosis of bilateral epidural hematoma. The patient next underwent bilateral craniotomies, with evacuation of large epidural clots (arterial source), and had a ventriculostomy placed. The child went to the pediatric ICU postoperatively, was moved 4 days later to the ward, and remained in the hospital for 7 additional days. His neurologic recovery was complete.

SUGGESTED READINGS

Eichelberger MR, Randolph JG: Pediatric trauma algorithm. *J Trauma* February 1983;23:91–97.

James HE, Anas NG, Perkin RM: *Brain Insults in Infants*. Orlando, FL, Grune & Stratton, 1985.

Raphaely RC, Swedlow DB, Downes JJ, et al: Management of severe pediatric head trauma. *Pediatr Clin North Am* 1980;27:714.

Case 43

Seven-year-old Male with Headache and Stiff Neck

CASE PRESENTATION

A 7-year-old male was sent to the emergency department by his local pediatrician for a lumbar puncture to rule out viral meningitis. Three days before arrival the child became sick and was described by his parents as being sleepy and taking multiple naps. During a visit to his pediatrician that day a CBC was performed and the diagnoses of anemia and sore throat were made. Cephalexin (Keflex®) was prescribed. The child described two short episodes of double vision while watching television on the 2 days preceding arrival in the emergency department. He complained of an intermittent headache, which was treated with acetaminophen.

The child was seen again by his pediatrician because he was somewhat somnolent. On examination the child's neck was stiff. Because it was late summer the child was referred to rule out viral meningitis.

Vital Signs

T: 37.1°C (98.8°F)
P: 100 beats/min
RR: 20/min
BP: 104/70 mm Hg
WT: 24.8 kg

Physical Examination

GEN: Alert, happy, talkative child in no distress
HEENT: *Eyes:* PERRLA; EOM intact; bilateral papilledema of fundi. *Ears:* normal eardrums. *Nose:* clear. *Throat:* negative
NECK: Full active range of motion without pain; however, when the neck was hyperflexed by the examiner the child screamed and cried in pain
CHEST: Clear to palpation and auscultation
CVS: Regular rhythm; no murmur
ABD: Soft; no organomegaly
GU: Normal circumcised prepubertal male
NEURO: Normal gait: equal muscle strength in upper and lower extremities; reflexes +1 in upper extremities and ankles, +2 at knees; downgoing toes

SUGGESTED INTERVENTIONS

1. Start IV with normal saline at strict KVO.
2. Obtain blood specimens for CBC, differential, glucose, and ESR.
3. Keep patient NPO.
4. Order CT scan of brain with and without contrast media.
5. Perform lumbar puncture only if CT scan is negative for mass lesion or increased pressure.
6. Consider admission.

CASE DISCUSSION

Nuchal rigidity and headache in children results most frequently from either viral or bacterial meningitis. The relatively infrequent occurrences of other causes may lead the physician to omit portions of the physical examination or neglect considering a complete differential diagnostic list.

Bacterial meningitis most commonly affects children below age 5 with the peak below age 2½ years. The children are almost always febrile and irritable, especially when gently shaken. Seizures and extreme lethargy are alternate presentations. Meningitis does not reliably produce a stiff neck in children under 18 months of age; therefore, absence of a stiff neck in no way rules out meningitis in this age-group.

A funduscopic examination should be performed on all children and infants about to undergo lumbar puncture for suspected meningitis. To examine an infant, who will tend to fix on the ophthalmoscopic light, the examiner holds the instrument in a fixed location aimed at the usual location of the disk. The child will eventually tire of watching the light and allow his eyes to roam. While the eye is moving the disk will move through the examiner's field of vision.

Viral meningitis may affect any age and is most frequently seen during the summer. There is often a "flu" prodrome followed by fever in nearly all children. Young children exhibit the nonspecific symptoms of lethargy, vomiting, diarrhea, rash, or GI symptoms. The older child will be lethargic, complain of headache and photophobia, and may vomit. Although this disease is usually mild, younger infants may develop seizures or apnea. Lumbar puncture confirms the diagnosis, but the relative risks of a "tap" in a patient with a possible intracranial mass lesion must be entertained.

The differential diagnostic list also includes subarachnoid bleeding from vascular abnormalities. These patients usually have sudden onset of severe headache and stiff neck caused by meningeal irritation by blood. Patients may progress rapidly or slowly into coma, or they may remain somewhat somnolent and complain of continuous headache. If the bleeding occurs in the parenchyma, the child may experience seizures or exhibit gross neurologic deficits. Small children are most likely to present with seizures, focal neurologic deficits, or general irritability rather than simple coma. When subarachnoid bleeding is suspected, a CT scan should be performed. If the patient develops impending herniation, then intubation, hyperventilation, and therapy with dexamethasone and mannitol should be used to reverse the increased pressure.

Brain tumors, particularly those in the posterior fossa, may cause increased pressure resulting in cerebellar tonsillar herniation with compression of the brain stem. The headache usually precedes the nuchal rigidity for a few days to months. The headache is usually worse in the morning and may wake the child and/or be accompanied by vomiting and ataxia. Vomiting alone may be the only symptom. Fever is extremely unusual. The complaint of diplopia strongly suggests cranial nerve compression. Papilledema is a late finding. A CT scan should be obtained in any child with any suggestion of posterior fossa tumor.

Nuchal rigidity is also seen in poliomyelitis and leptospirosis. Spinal cord tumors and transverse myelopathy produce stiff neck but usually not headache.

Infections of the pharynx such as peritonsillar abscess, retropharyngeal abscess, and cervical lymphadenitis all produce limited neck mobility. Torticollis often accompanies retropharyngeal abscess, may be traumatic, or may occur completely de novo. ESR elevation may be the only hematologic abnormality seen in these inflammatory entities. Lateral soft tissue films of the neck are excellent aids to these diagnoses.

Morquio's syndrome, juvenile rheumatoid arthritis, and Down's syndrome may be associated with subluxation of C1 on C2, with resulting pain and torticollis. A full cervical spine series with open mouth views is necessary to evaluate these children.

Discitis most frequently affects the lumbar spine but may involve the neck. The WBC count and ESR may be elevated, the disk space widened, and the bone scan positive in this disease. Fever is usually present.

In general, the initial "emergent" workup of stiff neck and headache aims to separate meningitis from intracranial masses and/or bleeding, as well as locating structural or inflammatory neck lesions. The history of trauma, or the presence of fever, mass, or neurologic abnormality, narrows the diagnostic possibilities.

This child had early morning lethargy, diplopia, and headache preceding a stiff neck by 3 days. The presence of papilledema strongly suggested increased intracranial pressure. A CT scan of the brain revealed a large tumor in the right posterior parietal lobe with extension to the right occipital and temporal lobe plus the thalamus. The child was admitted to the ICU and begun on dexamethasone, 1 mg/kg, with resolution of his symptoms within 24 hours.

SUGGESTED READINGS

Allen JC: Childhood brain tumors: Current status of clinical trials in newly diagnosed and recurrent disease. *Pediatr Clin North Am* 1985;32:633.

Doughty RA: Stiff neck. In Fleisher GR, Ludwig S (eds.): *Textbook of Pediatric Emergency Medicine*. Baltimore, Williams & Wilkins, 1983, pp. 194–197.

Walker RW, Allen JC: Pediatric brain tumors. *Pediatr Ann* 1983;12:383.

Seven-and-one-half-year-old Male with Head Injury, Headache, and Hemophilia A

CASE PRESENTATION

A 7½-year-old white male known to have hemophilia A diagnosed at birth with continuous bleeding at his circumcision site was brought to the emergency department.

His current illness began on the morning of admission when he hit his head on a sharp edge of a kitchen cabinet. He struck his right temporal area and sustained no loss of consciousness but had a persistent headache. He was perfectly oriented to time and place. There was no neurologic symptomatology by history, but he was nauseated without vomitus.

His most recent emergency department visit was 3 weeks prior to this presentation, at which time he was thought to have a soft tissue hematoma in the right forearm. He was treated with Factor VIII and had prompt resolution without compartment syndrome or other complications. No inhibitors were found. His hepatitis panels have been consistently negative, and he was HTLV-III negative, with good T4/T8 ratios.

Vital Signs

BP: 95/60 mm Hg
P: 85 beats/min (regular)
RR: 18/min
T: 37°C (98.6°F)
WT: 25 kg

Physical Examination

HEENT: *Head:* large subcutaneous hematoma in the right temporal fossa area. *Eyes:* PERRLA; EOM intact; normal fundi; no raccoon's eyes. *Ears:* normal tympanic membranes without hemotympanum; no Battle's sign. *Oropharynx:* normal

NECK: Supple; full range of motion; normal trachea; no stridor; no neck vein distention; no nodes

CHEST: Clear; normal to auscultation, percussion, and palpation; no evidence of rib fracture

CVS: Regular rhythm; no gallop rhythm, murmur, or rub; normal S_1 and S_2

ABD: Soft; nontender; no guarding; no costovertebral angle tenderness; no mass; no rebound; no liver, kidney, or spleen palpable; no flank hematoma

GU: *Rectum:* nontender; heme-negative stool

EXT: No acute swelling; all joints normal; old right forearm hematoma resolved without evidence for compartment swelling; all distal pulses strong and equal

NEURO: Alert; oriented to time, space, and self; complaining of bad headache; normoreflexive; normal cranial nerves, cerebellum, motor, and sensory examination; proprioception by gross testing; no clonus; no pathologic reflexes; Babinski's sign bilaterally plantar

SKIN: Old bruising; no acute bleeding

SUGGESTED INTERVENTIONS

1. Start IV with normal saline at KVO.
2. Obtain blood specimens for CBC, prothrombin time, and partial thromboplastin time, with 1:1 correction, and type and cross-match. Order urinalysis.
3. Administer Factor VIII, heat stabilized, 50 units/kg, or 1,250 units, stat IVSD.
4. Request stat neurosurgical consultation.
5. Order head CT scan without contrast media.
6. Admit the patient for neurologic observation and continued administration of Factor VIII.

CASE DISCUSSION

Classic hemophilia is a sex-linked recessive disease passed usually from mother to son. The incidence ranks approximately one case per 10,000 white male births.

The disease results from decreased Factor VIII activity in the presence of adequate Factor VIII antigen. This activity is generally reduced below 1% of normal in the seriously affected patient.

Serious sites of bleeding in the hemophiliac include retroperitoneal, in cases of abdominal and back trauma; retropharyngeal, in which case the enlarging hematoma encroaches on the airway; and intracranial bleeding, either spontaneous or in association with head trauma. The degree of trauma may be underestimated, and mistaken management follows. Any head injury sufficient to cause loss of consciousness, persistent nausea, vomiting, or headache should be treated immediately as life threatening. Intracranial bleeding is the leading (hemorrhagic) cause of death in these patients. The history cited in this case, with prolonged headache and nausea is enough for factor infusion, CT scanning, and admission for further observation and continued Factor VIII infusion. The additional risk factor of a temporal fossa injury overlying the thinnest portion of the temporal bone and the middle meningeal artery raises the probability of intracranial hemorrhage.

The blood initially obtained, after the IV line was established, was sent for routine CBC, type and cross-match (anticipating major hemorrhage), and prothrombin time and partial thromboplastin time. It takes a Factor VIII activity level of 40% or less to alter the partial thromboplastin time. Incubating the patient's plasma with normal plasma at a ratio of 1:1 (i.e., "1:1 correction") detects the presence of inhibitors to Factor VIII. Intubation with normal plasma should immediately correct the partial thromboplastin time abnormality of hemophilia A; however, if the patient has developed an inhibitor from prior transfusions of factor, this will inactivate the factor in normal plasma, and the partial thromboplastin time will not "correct."

Ten percent of hemophiliacs receiving Factor VIII will develop an IgG inhibitor to Factor VIII. There are "fast" responders who develop very high titers of inhibitors rapidly with exogenous factor. They quickly inactivate any additional infused factor. Corticosteroids and antineoplastic drugs such as cyclophosphamide have not proven to be effective in reducing this effect. In life-threatening situations with "fast" responders, exchange transfusion and massive Factor VIII infusion may save the patient. Other activated factor complexes such as Proplex® or Konÿne® can achieve hemostasis in these difficult patients.

"Slow" responders build up titer over several days after infusion, so generally Factor VIII that is infused is not destroyed before hemostasis is achieved.

This patient had a grossly abnormal partial thromboplastin time of 60 seconds but had a normal prothrombin time, CBC, and platelets. His 1:1 incubation corrected the partial thromboplastin time to normal, indicating absence of inhibitors.

This patient also had a benign neurologic examination. Nevertheless, his symptomatology indicated Factor VIII infusion, neurosurgical consultation, and mandatory CT scanning.

A hemophiliac on presentation should be considered to have no Factor VIII activity when seen. The object of Factor VIII infusion is to boost the activity level of Factor VIII to a percentage level considered adequate to correct the bleeding problem the patient has, or potentially has, such as suspected intracranial bleeding in this case. For bleeding into joints, soft tissue, or periarticular areas, a level of activity of 20% to 40% is targeted. For serious (potential) bleeding into the head or retropharyngeal or retroperitoneal areas, or for any surgical procedure (including suturing) 100% of activity is sought.

One unit per kilogram of Factor VIII will elevate the level of activity 2% (unless inhibitors are present). Therefore, for a target of 100% activity, 50 units/kg is infused. The half-life of this infused Factor VIII is 12 hours, so for admitted patients with potentially serious bleeding, such as this patient, the infusion of one-half the initial amount is continued every 12 hours (i.e., 25 units/kg).

The Factor VIII sources available include unconcentrated cold-precipitable fractions of human plasma (cryoprecipitate), as well as fresh, fresh frozen, or lyophilized plasma. Unconcentrated preparations are unsuitable for major hemorrhages and are reserved for minor bleeding episodes when concentrates are not available.

Concentrated preparations of Factor VIII, such as Hemofil®, antihemophiliac factor (AHF), Factorate®, Profilate®, Koate-HT® and Humafac®, have the advantages of smaller volume of infusant and a more standardized activity. They can be stored at 4°C and may be carried by the patients while traveling. They all carry the risk of hepatitis and, in porcine or bovine concentrates, the risk of allergic reaction.

The urinalysis came back 30 to 50 RBCs per high-powered field. For uncomplicated hematuria the patient should be started on prednisone, 2 mg/kg/day, when the CT scan is done, and the patient is no longer NPO. Isolated hematuria (in the absence of associated retroperitoneal or other serious hematoma) would be treated by infusing to a target of 40% to 50%. Epsilon-aminocaproic acid (EACA or Amicar®) is strictly contraindicated with hematuria. Amicar® has its best effect with isolated mouth bleeding, as in dental procedures.

A body CT scan would be an ideal way to diagnose retroperitoneal hematoma. Finding a hematoma would automatically indicate 100% target activity and admission for bed rest and careful observation. Uncomplicated hematuria can be managed as an outpatient, with the patient returning daily for infusion of Factor VIII and monitoring for disappearance of the hematuria. Daily dosing is the same as the initial dosage.

The neurosurgeon agreed that although there was no localizing findings or any suspicion of intracranial hemorrhage, the CT scan of the head was necessary. The scan was accomplished without contrast medium and was negative.

The patient was admitted and kept under observation. His symptoms resolved and he was discharged on the third day.

SUGGESTED READINGS

Eyster ME, Gill FM, Blatt PM, et al: CNS bleeding in hemophiliacs. *Blood* 1978;51:1179.

Jones P: Problems in the management of hemophilia. *Semin Hematol* 1977;14:375.

Lanzkowsky P: Hematologic emergencies. *Pediatr Clin North Am* 1979;26:909.

Eight-year-old Male with Vomiting, Lethargy, and Disorientation

CASE PRESENTATION

An 8-year-old white male presented with a 1-day history of vomiting. The emesis is nonbilious without associated fever, abdominal pain, or diarrhea. The mother states that he is lethargic and at times appears to be hallucinating. His past history is significant for a flulike illness 2 weeks ago. He is receiving no medications except aspirin, 160 mg, two or three times per day. There is no history of head trauma, pica, ingestion of foreign substances, seizures, or other neurologic problems. His development has been normal. He is currently on clear liquids. His urine output is reported as normal.

Vital Signs

T: 37°C (98.6°F)
HR: 110 beats/min
RR: 26/min
BP: 100/60 mm Hg
WT: 26 kg

Physical Examination

GEN: Lethargic, but arousable male
HEENT: *Head:* NCAT. *Eyes:* nonicteric sclera; clear conjunctiva; EOM intact; PERRLA; flat discs. *Ears:* normal tympanic membranes. *Oropharynx:* moist mucous membranes and no injection
NECK: Supple without adenopathy

CHEST: Clear to auscultation with no retractions
CVS: Regular rate and rhythm without S_3, S_4, or murmur; full pulses
ABD: Normoactive bowel sounds; liver 2 cm below the right costal margin and slightly tender; no palpable spleen or masses
GU: *Genitalia:* normal male. *Rectum:* normal
NEURO: Lethargic, but arousable; opens eyes spontaneously; spontaneous vocalizations; localizes pain and follows commands; intact cranial nerves; normal motor function, sensation, and coordination; normal reflexes with downgoing toes
SKIN: Acyanotic with good perfusion

SUGGESTED INTERVENTIONS

1. Place on cardiac monitor.
2. Administer oxygen, 3 L/min.
3. Obtain blood specimens for CBC, platelet count, electrolytes, BUN, creatinine, glucose, Dextrostix®, SGOT, bilirubin, ammonia, prothrombin time, partial thromboplastin time, salicylate level, toxicologic screen, amylase, type and cross-match, and ABGs.
4. Obtain urine specimen for urinalysis and toxicologic screen.
5. Establish an IV line with normal saline at strict KVO.
6. Administer naloxone (Narcan®), 0.01 mg/kg, IV—minimum, 1 ampule (0.4 mg).
7. Give 50% dextrose in water, 1–2 cc/kg IVp; Dextrostix® = 40 mg/dL.
8. Order CT scan of head, with and without contrast media.
9. Give vitamin K, 0.1 mg/kg, IM or slow IV if the prothrombin time is prolonged.
10. Infuse fresh frozen plasma if there is any evidence of bleeding.
11. Perform lumbar puncture. Defer procedure if CT scan suggests increased cerebral pressure or for any evidence of bleeding.
12. Admit patient to a pediatric ICU for close observation. Initiate full cerebral resuscitation for any disorientation (see discussion below).

CASE DISCUSSION

Reye's syndrome is a multisystem disease of unknown etiology characterized primarily by a progressive encephalopathy and fatty degeneration of the liver, but with mitochondrial degeneration in all tissues. It occurs seasonally with peaks of incidence occurring in December to March and June to July.

The illness is biphasic. Ninety percent of those affected have a history of an antecedent viral illness, especially influenza B and varicella. Usually the child is beginning to recover from the viral illness when there is an abrupt onset of vomiting without fever, diarrhea, or abdominal pain. This is followed in 24 to 48 hours by signs of encephalopathy. This encephalopathy may appear initially as lethargy or apathy but can progress to combativeness, agitation, disorientation, stupor, and coma. In infants under 1 year of age vomiting may be absent, with apnea, hypoglycemia, and seizures predominating clinically. Seizures are a late sign in older children.

On presentation to the emergency department the child is usually afebrile and often has tachycardia and tachypnea. The blood pressure is usually normal unless significant increased intracranial pressure is present. A mild degree of dehydration may be present secondary to vomiting and decreased oral intake. There is no evidence of jaundice, but hepatomegaly is present in about 50% of patients. Focal neurologic findings and meningismus are usually absent. The level of coma is an important prognostic factor and determinant of therapy. The stages have been described by Lovejoy as follows:

Stage I: The patient is vomiting and lethargic but follows commands.

Stage II: The patient is lethargic to stuporous and disoriented but with normal responses to pain and pupillary reflexes. Combativeness is noted.

Stage III: The patient is comatose with inappropriate responses to pain and decorticate posturing.

Stage IV: The patient is comatose with decerebrate posturing, loss of oculocephalic reflexes, disconjugate gaze, and dilated pupils.

Stage V: The patient is flaccid and apneic with no response to pain and no pupillary or oculocephalic reflexes.

The diagnosis of Reye's syndrome is based on the clinical presentation and laboratory evaluation. There are many conditions that may mimic Reye's syndrome especially in the early stages. In Reye's syndrome the SGOT, SGPT, and ammonia levels are almost always elevated. The bilirubin is greater than 2.0 mg/dL in only 10% of patients, which can be used to distinguish Reye's syndrome from fulminant hepatitis. The prothrombin time is prolonged in about 50% of patients, but the hemoglobin, hematocrit, and platelet count are usually normal. The BUN is elevated in 30% to 40% of patients, probably secondary to a mild dehydration. Hypoglycemia may be present, especially in children under 1 year of age. Many patients exhibit a high anion-gap acidosis with elevated lactic acid levels and a compensatory respiratory hyperventilation. Serum ketones, uric acid, and creatine phosphokinase levels may also be elevated. A salicylate level should be obtained not only because Reye's syndrome has been associated with the use of salicylates but also because Reye's syndrome and salicylate toxicity have very similar clinical and laboratory presentations. A drug screen is indicated to rule out toxic causes of metabolic encephalopathy such as lead and ethanol. A lumbar puncture is contraindicated during an acute spike in intracranial pressure but should be performed in most stage I patients to rule out meningitis and encephalitis. The CT scan of the head was used in this case to rule out occult trauma, intracerebral mass lesion, and suggestions of increased cerebral pressure. In the nonfebrile encephalopathic patient with closed fontanelles it is always safer to have a negative CT scan prior to lumbar puncture. Because the cerebral edema in Reye's syndrome is diffuse, complications of the spinal tap are rare. In Reye's syndrome the opening pressure is usually elevated, but the CSF protein, cell count, and Gram stain are normal. Further workup for possible inborn errors of metabolism (e.g., urea cycle disorders) should be undertaken after appropriate consultation.

Despite the generalized mitochondrial defect, morbidity and mortality are primarily determined by the degree of cerebral edema and increased intracranial pressure. All patients suspected of Reye's syndrome, even in the early stages, should be admitted to a pediatric intensive care unit not only because of the potential for rapid deterioration, but because good supportive care is critical in determining outcome.

Patients in stage I should be monitored every 15 minutes for vital signs and neurologic status. An IV of 10% dextrose in 0.3 normal saline at two thirds maintenance is indicated unless there is more than a mild (<5%) dehydration present. It is very important not to overhydrate the patient. If the patient is hypoglycemic, 50% dextrose at 1–2 mg/kg IV is indicated. Vitamin K and fresh frozen plasma are indicated for a prolonged prothrombin time and evidence of bleeding.

Patients with stages III to IV disease require full cerebral resuscitation. Invasive monitoring by a ventriculostomy or subarachnoid bolt, arterial line, and central venous pressure line is indicated. These patients require intubation, hyperventilation, paralysis, mannitol, and barbiturate coma, as well as full supportive care.

The treatment of patients with stage II disease is less clear. Most centers will manage these patients similar to those with stage I disease but will institute aggressive therapy if there is any deterioration.

There is a 15% to 30% overall mortality rate. The mortality and morbidity are greater in younger patients and also the more advanced the stage of coma on admission, so early recognition and hospitalization are imperative. Children over 1 year of age with stage I or II disease on admission generally do well with no significant neurologic sequelae.

Because of the association between salicylate ingestion and Reye's syndrome, the American Academy of Pediatrics recommends that salicylates not be given to children suspected of having varicella or influenza.

SUGGESTED READINGS

Bellman MH, Ross EM, Miller DL: Reye's syndrome in children under three years old. *Arch Dis Child* 1982;57:259.

Consensus Conference: Diagnosis and treatment of Reye's syndrome. *JAMA* 1981;246:2441.

Fleisher G, Ludwig S: *Textbook of Pediatric Emergency Medicine*. Baltimore, Williams and Wilkins, 1983, pp 567–572.

Lovejoy FH, Smith AL, Brennan MJ, et al: Clinical staging in Reye's syndrome. *Am J Dis Child* 1974;128:36.

Shaywitz SE, Cohen PM, Cohen DJ, et al: Long-term consequences of Reye's syndrome: A sibling matched controlled study of neurologic, cognitive, academic and psychiatric function. *J Pediatr* 1982;100:41.

Starko KM, Ray CG, Dominguez LB, et al: Reye's syndrome and salicylate use. *Pediatrics* 1980;66:859.

Trauner D: Management of Reye's syndrome. In James HE, Anas NG, Perkin RM (eds): *Brain Insults in Infants and Children*. Orlando, FL, Grune & Stratton, 1985, pp 216–220.

Case 46

Nine-year-old Male with Multiple Blunt Trauma, Hypotension, and Gross Hematuria

CASE PRESENTATION

A 9-year-old male ran across the street and was hit by an oncoming automobile traveling approximately 35 mph. The child was struck against his left pelvis by the front right bumper of the automobile and was subsequently thrown to the ground. He struck his left flank and left lower chest, and the impact was partially broken by his outstretched left hand. There was no immediate loss of consciousness; the child refused lower extremity movement but moved his neck spontaneously without pain to all observers.

The parents did not wait for the paramedics but scooped up the patient and brought him to the emergency department, carrying him in their arms. There were never any signs of external bleeding seen by the parents. The child remained awake and was moaning in mild distress on arrival.

The child's past medical history, quickly obtained from the mother, was essentially negative, with all immunizations current and no known drug allergies. There was no history of prior serious injury, burn, or ingestion of foreign substances.

Vital Signs

BP: 65/40 mm Hg
P: 155 beats/min (weak)
RR: 35/min
WT: 30 kg (estimated)

Physical Examination

GEN: Awake, but obviously distressed child, with multiple bruises, with no acute respiratory embarrassment

HEENT: *Head:* all facial bones intact. *Eyes:* PERRLA; EOM intact; normal fundi; no raccoon's eyes. *Ears:* no hemotympanum; no Battle's sign. *Nose:* nares clear of blood/fluid. *Oropharynx:* no oral lesions

NECK: Full spontaneous range of motion; nontender to palpation; no deformity or crepitance; midline trachea; no neck vein distention; no Kussmaul's sign

CHEST: Crepitant left lateral lower rib cage; no visible flail; decreased breath sounds in left chest, with tympanitic left hemothorax; + intracostal flaring; increased RR to 35/min, regular; anteroposterior/lateral compression tenderness referred to left lateral chest wall; subcutaneous emphysema noted along this portion of rib cage

CVS: Tachycardia; no gallop rhythm; no rub; (?) point of maximal impulse displaced to left parasternal area; S_1 slightly increased; no murmurs heard

ABD: Left upper quadrant tenderness with involuntary guarding; normal bowel sounds, no rebound; abdomen nondistended; no costovertebral angle tenderness; no flank bruise; large abrasion overlying the left upper quadrant

GU: *Rectum:* very tender prostatic fossa, boggy with ill-defined prostatic mass; palpable fracture of right inferior pubic ramus and ischial ramus transrectally; light brown stool; heme-negative; good sphincter tone. *Pelvis:* very tender to anteroposterior/lateral compression; appears stable; tenderness localized to right side of pubic and ischial areas; sacroiliac joints intact; obvious ecchymosis near right ischial tuberosity region. *Genitalia:* gross blood exuding from urethral meatus; tenderness with (?) hematoma at base of penis at bulbospongiosum; both testes descended and without tenderness, hematoma, or swelling; circumcised glans

EXT: All extremities without obvious dislocation or gross fracture; refuses movement of lower left extremity, referring pain to hip region; all extremities with normal motor/sensory/vascular status, except as noted above; positive "snuff box" tenderness of left wrist; no obvious deformity

NEURO: Awake; alert; Glasgow Coma Score of 15; all protective reflexes intact; motor/sensory/cranial nerves/cerebellum/posterior columns all intact; no clonus; no pathologic reflexes; tone normal throughout; normoreflexive

SKIN: Mottled; all areas slightly cool; ecchymoses of right perineum and left upper quadrant as indicated above; no cyanosis

SUGGESTED INTERVENTIONS

1. Administer oxygen, 5 L/min, via nasal prongs.
2. Needle left chest with No. 18 angiocath in anterior axillary line in approximate fourth or fifth intercostal space. Reassess lung findings after this procedure.
3. Place MAST suit under patient, with leg portions expanded immediately.
4. Insert two large-bore catheters in antecubital areas, hooked to lactated Ringer's, and run in under pressure until blood pressure normalizes (approximately 100 mm Hg systolic for a 9-year-old).
5. Place on cardiac monitor.
6. Obtain blood specimens stat for type and cross-match, whole blood, 6 to 8 units, CBC, and amylase determination.
7. Insert NG tube to low continuous suction, Hematest®; irrigate until clear if grossly bloody.
8. Splint left wrist.
9. Order stat semiupright chest film and supine pelvic film. Patient must be kept supine for chest film if blood pressure has not normalized with volume infusion.
10. Expand abdominal portion of MAST suit if blood pressure has not normalized with volume infusion. Delay this if possible until a surgeon sees the patient.
11. Perform retrograde urethrogram with Conray-30®, under fluoroscopic observation if patient is stable (otherwise with portable technique in trauma room). If urethra is patent, pass Foley catheter into bladder; if urethra is disrupted, a suprapubic tube is placed by urologist or general surgeon. A No. 14 angiocath may be placed, as in a suprapubic tap, to divert urine, and monitor urine output if surgical consultation is much delayed. This is a temporizing procedure.
12. Order a body CT scan with pelvic cuts, with contrast media, if patient is stable enough to go to scan suite, or, if still hemodynamically unstable, peritoneal lavage (preferably after surgeon has evaluated abdomen), followed by "emergency" infusion intravenous pyelography, using 2 mL/kg (60 mL) of Renograffin-60®, with scout abdomen, and films at 5, 10, and 20 minutes (if still in emergency department). Following visualization of kidney and ureters, a cystogram is obtained using 10 mL/kg (300 mL) of

Conray-30®, instilled through the Foley catheter or suprapubic tube, which is clamped and followed by obtaining views of the bladder.
13. Admit the patient to the general pediatric service.

CASE DISCUSSION

This 9-year-old male was the victim of a high-speed pedestrian versus automobile accident that initially impacted him on his left side and threw him to the ground on his left side. There was no manifest craniocervical injury, nor was there a history of loss of consciousness. However, the patient presented to the emergency department without the benefit of a prehospital intervention and was hypotensive and in moderate respiratory distress. He refused motion of his left lower extremity, had obvious left chest and left upper abdominal injuries, and had a very suggestive left navicular wrist fracture. Equally distressing was the gross blood coming from his urethral meatus, and most signs and symptoms pointed to a fractured pelvis with concomitant urethral disruption, most likely at the prostatic urethra.

We generally insist on rigid cervical spine precautions in multiple trauma victims until the status of the bony cervical spine is determined. However, this patient was observed to move his neck in all ranges of motion without any pain or restriction and his initial emergency department evaluation showed a completely normal spine, without pain, deformity, or crepitance.

Initial primary survey and resuscitative efforts, directed at stabilizing the "ABCs" (airway, breathing, and circulation), consisted of starting oxygen immediately via nasal prongs and needling the chest to rule out significant pneumothorax (either simple or under tension). Although the trachea was not deviated, the patient was in respiratory distress, with hypotension, shifted mediastinum, and tympanitic left chest with absent breath sounds. This was not an indication to do a chest x-ray. It was essential to rule out these two possibilities immediately, and a needle thoracocentesis, done in the lateral approach, is our preferred route. The absence of neck vein distention does not rule out the possibility of tension pneumothorax, since the patient may have also been hypovolemic from hemorrhage either in the chest or elsewhere. This principle applies for pericardial tamponade as well, where a patient does not have enough circulating blood volume to manifest neck vein distention. Traumatologists also make a point of how similar left-sided tension pneumothorax and pericardial tamponade can mimic each other, with quiet heart sounds, shock, and frequently distended neck veins. The probability of this patient having pericardial tamponade with blunt lateral chest trauma was small.

With needle thoracocentesis air was noted to escape but not under pressure, and his respiratory rate improved but not back to normal. His breath sounds were heard much better on the left, and his point of maximal impulse was now in the normal apical position. His blood pressure came up slightly, but finally normalized to 100 mm Hg systolic after 600 mL of Ringer's lactate was infused (approximately 20 mL/kg), at which time his pulse returned to a normal of 85 beats/min.

We insist on two large lines (minimum) for multiple trauma with unstable hemodynamic presentation, and 16-gauge angiocaths should be considered for a 9-year-old. The largest diameter possible should be used! We do not hook up Pedidrips® for trauma and similarly do not use pediatric extension tubing, since these narrow diameters make rapid infusion of crystalloid or blood impossible. There is no rationale for central venous pressure monitoring initially in trauma resuscitation; it may be very useful subsequently, but initially they usually take too long to place. Two peripheral large-bore catheters in the antecubital veins is the best way to start. If lines are difficult at the onset, one team must be assigned to initiate cutdown or percutaneous access to a large vein. Our favorites are the basilic vein at the distal medial humerus, the femoral vein at the groin (good for percutaneous or cutdown on the saphenofemoral at the fossa ovale), the external jugular vein (if neck trauma ruled out), and finally the percutaneous internal jugular or subclavian veins. Procedures using these latter two veins take the most skill but in expert hands can be performed in less than 1 minute, with low complication rates, similar to adult experience.

The use of the MAST suit must be emphasized in the acute trauma pediatric patient presenting with hypotension. Initially, inflating the leg portion may elevate the peripheral resistance enough to begin perfusing other essential beds, such as the cardiac, renal, cerebral, and splanchnic, while attempts are being made to start lines. There is a small internal "transfusion" effect, but the best effect is its augmentation of resistance and decrease in venous capacitance. They are marvelous for stabilizing lower extremity fractures and can tamponade serious bleeding (external) in the lower extremities. Much is written about its salutary effect on stabilizing and tamponading intractable hemorrhage from serious pelvic fractures with large pelvic hematomas. However, this necessitates the abdominal compartment being inflated, so we try to delay this until the surgeon has evaluated the abdomen and a decision about peritoneal lavage is made. However, in profound exsanguinating hemorrhage (from the chest, abdomen, pelvis, or extremities) all portions of the MAST suit must be inflated on first presentation. After severe shock it must not be deflated until in the secure environment of surgery or intensive care, with appropriate prealkalinization and volume replacement. There are too many stories of sudden arrest simultaneous with MAST suit deflation for this to be undertaken lightly.

Blood secured with initial venipunctures must be sent for type and cross-match. Our general guideline is for any multiple trauma with obvious or suspected life-threatening hemorrhage, we type and cross-match initially for at least 100% of total blood volume (TBV); since TBV = (approximately) 8% of a child's weight, and we estimated this child to be 30 kg, an appropriate initial type and cross-match would have been for $30,000 \times 0.08 = 2,400$ mL of whole blood. This would be 5 units. This guideline is a minimum and could be expanded to 150% to 200% depending on suspicions and initial presentation. Since this child presented hypotensive and had many reasons to be in hemorrhagic shock, the initial type and cross-match was for 150% replacement, or 8 units. The mistake too often made in cases of multiple trauma is ordering blood too little and/or too late.

The CBC is helpful but only to compare with subsequent CBCs. As a guideline we repeat CBCs (or at least the hematocrit) every 30 to 45 minutes that a multiple trauma patient is in our emergency department. Remember the usual child's hematologic response to acute hemorrhage is the following: first a slight rise in hematocrit, then a rise in the WBC count, then finally a fall in hematocrit. The time course of these events is so variable that one must not rely on absolutes but must rather look at trends, and a falling hematocrit and a rising WBC are usually ominous. Delays of 2 to 3 hours until the hematocrits fall significantly are not unheard of with acute hemorrhage.

The amylase is only fairly sensitive to pancreatic injury, with many false negatives, but curiously there is a high correlation between a high amylase level and some serious injury in acute blunt abdominal trauma (although not necessarily pancreatic). We never rely on amylase values to dictate intervention, so in fact this test could be deleted.

The NG tube is essential in the child with multiple trauma. It must not be placed until the status of the cervical spine is ensured, since neck manipulation is required. Similarly, in a patient without a gag reflex the airway must be secured by intubation before the passage of the NG tube, since vomiting and aspiration could be a complication of passing the tube. Insertion of the tube is mandatory because of several important principles. All children who sustain trauma (either isolated or multiple) develop gastric atony very readily and very early. This compromises respiration and ultimately leads to vomiting and perhaps fatal aspiration. It is also useful to test the aspirated stomach contents for the presence of blood or bile. The displacement of the tube on plain films sometimes indicates splenic enlargement. The tube passage creates peristaltic waves, which may increase the amount of free air escaping a penetrated hollow viscus and cause it to appear earlier on upright or decubitus plain films. The tube should be aspirated and any contents checked by Gastroccult® for occult blood. If associated ingestion of a foreign substance is suspected to have precipitated the trauma, appropriate toxologic tests can be done on the gastric aspirant, the stomach can be lavaged, and charcoal can be instilled.

If gross blood appears, the tube should be irrigated with cool or iced saline until clear. The nostrils are checked for associated (iatrogenic) epistaxis. The tube should be hooked to low continuous Gomco® suction and appropriate intake and output notes made on this drainage.

After all stabilizing resuscitative procedures and surveys are completed the primary phase of resuscitation is completed. By this point any abnormality in the "ABCs" must be corrected, and all appropriate lines started and tubes placed.

The secondary phase of trauma assessment and management consists of a total head to toe reexamination of the patient, examining every orifice in a search for injuries missed on the rapid primary ("life-threat") survey. It is during this secondary phase that stat x-ray films are first ordered. This is a very important point, because in reality there is no reason to x-ray a patient until the life-threatening priorities are stabilized. If there is any suspicion of a tension pneumothorax, for instance, then the chest is needled. There is no time to wait for an x-ray. Any suspicious neck injury should automatically be stabilized, and the other life-threatening injuries managed.

There are only three stat portable x-ray views worth considering during the secondary phase of trauma survey and management in the trauma suite: the lateral cervical spine view, the upright chest view, and the anteroposterior pelvic view. The cervical spine should always be cleared in any patient who manifests neck pain, immobility, or deformity or who is too inebriated or lethargic to manifest these symptoms. In these patients a good lateral view, down to and including the vertebral body at the C7 level, is mandatory. A good technique that virtually ensures an adequate film is to have one assistant (wearing a shielded apron) pull down on the patient's wrists (assuming no fractures) while a second assistant (similarly shielded) applies countertraction against the patient's chin in an upward, cephalad direction. The summation of these forces effectively depresses the shoulders and almost always gets a good lateral film usually down to the T1 level and occasionally to T2. This patient had no signs or symptoms of cervical injury and was wide awake so a cervical spine film was not needed.

The chest film should be done as upright as possible depending on the patient's blood pressure. In this manner even small pneumothoraces can be seen. The chest film, especially an upright one, gives a wealth of information for the trauma patient: it defines cardiothoracic pathology, confirms tube and line position, may demonstrate free air under the diaphragm, and defines fractured ribs, which may themselves suggest other likely visceral injuries. A patient who is known to be hypotensive should not be put in an upright position since this may cause cardiac arrest. Also, in a normotensive patient it is wise to measure the pulse and blood pressure while sitting them up for the x-ray. The physician should look for subtle changes that may be suggestive of hemorrhage.

The pelvic x-ray is useful in most multiple trauma, even with much less suspicion of pelvic fracture than in the case presented here. This is a commonly missed fracture in childhood trauma, and the more pelvic films are ordered in the trauma suite, the more fractures will be found. A fractured pelvis is highly associated with copious and continuous bleeding, accounting for prolonged "occult" shock, or unexplained fall in the hematocrit. The early diagnosis can lead to earlier management, such as MAST suit tamponade, external skeletal fixation and arteriographic embolization, and occasionally surgery to control intractable bleeding. A ruptured bladder and urethra associated with the fragments of the bony pelvis may be missed because the pelvis was inadequately evaluated.

In this patient the chest film revealed that the left side of the chest was now completely evacuated of air and there was no apparent hemothorax. However, there was a fracture of the left lateral aspect of the 9, 10, and 11th ribs, with some subcutaneous emphysema. The heart size was normal. There was a questionable small left-sided pulmonary contusion.

The pelvic plain film revealed what was suspected clinically—that there were fractures of the right superior ramus and right ischiopubic ramus. There was a large soft tissue mass, suggesting pelvic hematoma.

The patient was very stable hemodynamically at this point, and with the agreement of the consulting surgeon, he was moved to the x-ray suite where a retrograde urethrogram was done showing disruption at the prostatic urethra. The surgeon placed a Bonano suprapubic catheter to drain urine and measure urine output.

The patient next had an abdominal CT scan with cuts of the pelvis. This study is always done with contrast infusion. If it is done following a head CT scan, the head is scanned without contrast and then the abdominal scan is done with contrast. The abdominal scan in our patient showed a small subcapsular splenic hematoma but normal pancreas, kidneys, ureter, liver, and bladder. There was a small right-sided pelvic hematoma associated with obvious bone fragments, as indicated above. There was no apparent large retroperitoneal hematoma seen.

The use of abdominal CT scanning in patients stable enough to go to the CT suite has increased our sensitivity to lesions in solid viscera and aided our assessment of hematoma presence and size. It has proven ideal for the assessment of the pelvis and pelvic hematoma. It retains very little diagnostic acumen for hollow viscus perforation, but when combined with plain films, and Gastrograffin® swallow (not indicated in this patient), intestinal perforations and intramural hematomas may be demonstrated.

If we are unable to take the child to the CT suite because of hemodynamic instability, we do as much of the workup as possible in the trauma room, evacuating the child to surgery as soon as possible. If intra-abdominal crisis is obvious and the patient is unstable, no lavage of the peritoneum is done: this is an obvious surgical candidate. If there are equivocal abdominal findings, with instability, a lavage is done. The bladder and stomach should be appropriately intubated and decompressed first, and an infraumbilical approach is used, with direct vision of the linea alba and penetration with a peritoneal dialysis catheter. If there is a suspicion of pelvic fracture and hematoma, then a supraumbilical approach is recommended.

The catheter is immediately aspirated, and bright blood, or obvious intestinal contents, constitute a positive tap. Otherwise 10 to 15 mL/kg of lactated Ringer's is infused and then allowed to dwell in the abdomen for several minutes while the patient is log-rolled from side to side. The fluid is gravity drained and sent for CBC, amylase determination, and Gram stain and dipped for bile. A CBC over 100,000 RBCs per high-powered field or positive bile or bacteria or an elevated amylase level all indicate positivity. The false-positive and false-negative rates in most studies are each 1% to 2%.

If the child must go urgently to surgery, then a 2 mL/kg intravenous pyelogram done either in the emergency department or immediately on arrival in the operating room will help define the status of the kidneys. Similarly the retrograde urethrogram and cystogram can be deferred to the operating room and be done with a urologist present.

This patient stabilized fairly readily, and we elected to observe both splenic and pelvic hematomas, leaving the abdominal MAST suit in place. He was next taken to the ICU. X-ray films of the left wrist revealed a navicular fracture, which was immobilized in a thumb spica cast by an orthopedist.

He recovered from all of his injuries, including the urethral tear, which also was managed nonoperatively with a small stent catheter. He left the hospital on the 12th day and is recovering well.

SUGGESTED READINGS

Eichelberger MR, Randolph JG: Pediatric trauma algorithm. *J Trauma* February 1983;23:91–97.

Haller JA, Reichard SA, Shorter N, et al: Pelvic fractures in children—a review of 120 cases. *J Pediatr Surg* 1980;15:727.

Morse TS: The child with multiple injuries. *Emerg Clin North Am* April 1983;1:175.

Thirteen-year-old Male with Limp and Pain in Left Leg

CASE PRESENTATION

A 13-year-old obese black male came to the emergency department in May complaining of a limp and pain in his mid left leg. He stated it was difficult to localize the pain, but it seemed to be mostly around this knee. He also thought his buttock ached at times. He first noted mild discomfort beginning about 2 weeks previously. The pain slowly increased in intensity during the 2 weeks but was not incapacitating. He did not remember any specific traumatic episode but he was active in sports.

There were no fevers, immunizations, viral illnesses, constitutional symptoms, weight loss, or medications for the past months.

The past medical history consisted of up-to-date immunizations and no serious illnesses or hospitalizations. The patient had been tested for sickle cell anemia and had neither the trait nor the disease.

Vital Signs

HR: 75 beats/min
RR: 16/min
BP: 120/75 mm Hg
T: 37.3°C (99.1°F)
WT: 60 kg (90th percentile)
HT: 145 cm (10th percentile)

Physical Examination

GEN: Well-appearing male with moderate obesity

HEENT: *Head:* NCAT. *Eyes:* PERRLA; EOM intact; conjunctiva clear. *Ears:* normal tympanic membranes. *Throat:* normal

NECK: Supple; shotty nodes

CHEST: Clear to palpation and auscultation

CVS: Regular rhythm; no murmur

ABD: Normal bowel sounds; no masses or organomegaly

GU: Normal circumcised male, Tanner stage II

EXT: Antalgic gait with the foot externally rotated on the left; examination of the hips revealed the following:

	Right (cm)	Left (cm)
Flexion	160	130
Extension	30	40
Internal rotation	60	20
External rotation	60	80
Abduction	20	15
Abduction	60	40
Leg length	71	69

There was pain on extreme flexion and internal rotation on the left. There also was discomfort on palpation of anterior aspect of hip capsule but no erythema or warmth around hips. Examination of knees and ankles was normal.

SUGGESTED INTERVENTIONS

1. Keep patient non-weight-bearing.
2. Order anteroposterior and true lateral (Clayton-Johnson) views of left hip.
3. Request orthopedic consultation.
4. Admit patient for traction and surgical stabilization.

CASE DISCUSSION

A slipped capital femoral epiphysis is an easy diagnosis to make once the possibility is considered. The disorder affects children just before or during their adolescent growth spurt. It should be pointed out that the growth spurt begins before the onset of sexual maturation, which means girls are at risk for the disease from age 8 to 15 and boys from age 10 to 17. Facts associated with increased risk include male sex, black race, obese stature, delayed bone age, and the spring or summer months.

Occasionally the capital epiphysis can slip acutely both during birth or during late adolescence. In these cases major trauma is necessary and the child has severe pain and inability to walk.

Much more commonly the slip is slowly progressive and the process may proceed for months before the diagnosis is made. Since the outcome is strongly related to degree of slip, the diagnosis must be made early. A history of trauma is rarely present.

The patient usually limps and keeps the foot externally rotated. The pain may be very mild to severe and may affect the hip, anterior thigh, buttocks, or knee. As a rule, knee pain in children should always lead to examination of the hip as well as the knee.

The examination of the hip begins with measurement of leg length from anterior-superior iliac spine to the medial malleolus. Hip disease usually leads to shortening of the affected leg. The circumference of the thighs 2 inches superior to the patellae and of the calves at their largest portion is measured. Chronic pain will lead to decreased use of the extremity and atrophy of the muscles.

Next, the range of motion at the hips is recorded and compared from side to side. Luckily, most persons have a normal joint on the opposite side to which the range of motion in the abnormal side can be compared. Difference between sides means there is a pathologic problem. When the capital epiphysis slips, internal rotation, abduction, and flexion are all limited at the hip.

These specific motions are limited because the femoral head usually slips posterior and medially off the femoral neck. With the femoral head slipped into this position, it occupies a position in the acetabulum corresponding to partial internal rotation, abduction, and flexion. Likewise, the patient must externally rotate the foot during ambulation in order to move the abnormal inwardly rotated head into the neutral position.

Palpation of the joint capsule and pelvis should be carried out. Likewise, warmth, erythema, or swelling of the joint should be sought.

In patients who present with knee pain, the knee should be examined, including range of motion, ligament and semilunar cartilage integrity, patellar function, and tibial tubercle tenderness. The presence of fluid or other signs of inflammation is also noted.

An anteroposterior and true lateral (Clayton-Johnson) view of the affected hip should be taken. The true lateral view reveals a slight degree of posterior slip much more clearly than the frog-leg lateral view. Therefore, the diagnosis in early disease is less likely to be missed. Obviously once a slip is entertained, the child should be kept non-weight-bearing until after the x-ray film confirms or refutes the diagnosis.

The differential diagnosis becomes important only after the x-ray films rule out slipped epiphysis. Low-grade infection such as tuberculosis should be considered. Toxic synovitis, monoarticular juvenile rheumatoid arthritis, osteochondritis dissecans, idiopathic chondrolysis, and late-onset Legg Perthes avascular necrosis of the femoral head should all be considered. A CBC and ESR may be helpful in inflammatory diseases. A bone scan may be abnormal in Legg-Perthes disease and osteochondritis dissecans.

The patient with a slipped epiphysis should be admitted for traction and eventual stabilization of the slipping femoral head. In cases of advanced slipping, various osteotomies are used to realign the joint.

SUGGESTED READINGS

Chung S: Diseases of the developing hip joint. *Pediatr Clin North Am* 1977;24:857.

Neinstein LS: *Adolescent Health Care: A Practical Guide.* Baltimore, Urban and Schwarzenberg, 1984, pp 191–192.

Case 48

Fourteen-year-old Female with Facial Pain and Agitation

CASE PRESENTATION

A 14-year-old female was brought to the emergency department complaining of facial pain on the right side. The symptoms were present when she awoke that morning and progressed throughout the morning. During the first 15 minutes she became increasingly upset and complained more and more about the pain, which eventually also involved the same side of the neck. She became tearful and quite upset. Both she and her mother, who had remained in the room, denied any previous similar symptoms. They deny trauma of any kind and the use of any medications. There also were no associated symptoms. A second attempt to discuss possible drug use was cut short by the mother who exclaimed, "My child would never use any drugs."

The mother was excused from the room, and after a very tearful breakdown, the patient admitted taking four chlorpromazine (Thorazine®) capsules (belonging to her mother) in despondency over a failed romance. She had taken them 16 hours prior to arrival to the emergency department. The patient was very well oriented but seemed depressed. Reality testing was normal. The patient began having dysarthric symptoms at this point and further history taking was deferred.

Vital Signs

HR: 90 beats/min
RR: 16/min
BP: 110/75 mm Hg
T: 37.3°C (99.1°F)
WT: 85 kg
HT: 163 cm

Physical Examination

HEENT: *Head:* slight asymmetry with face muscles more tense on left; no increase in pain with palpation of left side of face; no redness or swelling. *Eyes:* PERRLA; EOM intact; normal fundi, with sharp disks; ? end-gaze nystagmus. *Ears:* normal. *Nose:* clear. *Oropharynx:* normal except patient seems to have difficulty opening her mouth

NECK: Initially full range of motion, although looking to left seemed to increase the neck pain

CHEST: Clear to auscultation

CVS: Regular rate and rhythm

ABD: Soft; normal bowel sounds; no masses or organomegaly

NEURO: Normal affect; normal associations; seemed depressed; moved all extremities. The remainder of the examination was difficult to perform because the patient became agitated. During the examination the patient's head rotated to the right and tilted upward into a fixed position. The examiner was unable to move the head to neutral, and attempts to do this caused an increase in pain. Rotatory nystagmus was observed. Reflexes seemed all 1 + and symmetric. There was no clonus. Babinski's sign was plantar. No pathologic reflexes elicited

SKIN: Clear

SUGGESTED INTERVENTIONS

1. Administer diphenhydramine, 50 mg, IM, or benztropine, 2 mg IM.
2. Order toxicologic screen of blood and urine, CBC, glucose determination, and Dextrostix® (result = 80 to 120 mg/dL).
3. After dystonia resolves, request psychosocial consultation with on-call psychiatrist to decide risk potential, appropriate admission or referral, and need for acute intervention.

CASE DISCUSSION

Phenothiazines cause several types of extrapyramidal side effects. Dystonic reactions, akathisia, and pseudoparkinsonism are idiosyncratic and not dose related and respond to benztropine, 2 mg, IM, or diphenhydramine (Benadryl®), 1.5 mg/kg, IM or IV. These reactions are caused by acute blocking of dopaminergic centers in the CNS, allowing cholinergic domination of central pathways, particularly in the extrapyramidal tracts. Since antihistamines are fairly potent anticholinergics, this explains the use of diphenhydramine in reversing the reaction. Benztropine, which has benzhydryl radicals (similar to diphenhydramine) and atropinic moieties (strongly anticholinergic), has proven superior to diphenhydramine for reversing this type of reaction. We generally do not use benztropine in children under 6 years of age. Tardive dyskinesia on the other hand results from long-term therapy and may not reverse. Children are more likely to develop these side effects. Additionally, children also can develop more severe reactions, including laryngospasm, tetanus-like syndromes, coma, apnea, and death. At least one study reported an increased incidence of sudden infant death syndrome in infants given phenothiazines as cough suppressants. The overall adverse reaction rate in children is 33% to 50%. Taking this into account the prudent emergency department physician will avoid the use of these medications in children. Because of its popularity as an antiemetic, prochlorperazine (Compazine®) accounts for a large number of these reactions.

Because the latency period may be long between administration and reaction there may be difficulty in eliciting a history of drug use. In addition, many parents simply do not consider these medications worth mentioning and the physician must ask directly about tranquilizers and antiemetics. Also, children may take these medications unobserved by an adult.

Adolescents *must* be interviewed alone. The physician in this case erred in allowing this patient's mother into the room. Allowing a parent to witness the history taking is an invasion of the teenage patient's privacy and will compromise the adolescent's honesty when answering sensitive questions. Once inaccurate information is stated, the patient will feel compelled to stick to the story regardless of whether the parent is present or absent.

Suicide is the leading cause of death in the teenage years. Often these adolescents have had a chaotic childhood followed by further isolation from their parents as they reach the teen years. The breakup of a significant relationship might trigger a suicide attempt. There are many myths about suicide. It is easiest to dispel them all with the statement that all suicidal attempts indicate a serious and potentially fatal situation requiring skilled assessment in the emergency department by a mental health provider who can assess the degree of risk.

Some of the areas addressed during the assessment include the following:

1. The ability of the patient to relate positively to the assessor. For this reason it is wise to avoid unpleasant comments to the patient regarding the suicide attempt.
2. The presence or absence of supportive parents who demonstrate empathy with the teen
3. The patient's feelings about being rescued, showing whether an ongoing degree of helplessness is present
4. The presence of previous attempts
5. The use of drugs or alcohol as a confounding factor

6. The degree of seriousness of this attempt (a few pills versus massive over-dose discovered accidentally)
7. If the patient is to be discharged, can the patient control his or her behavior until seen by a mental health care provider?

This patient's dystonia and dysarthria cleared in 45 minutes. Her toxicologic studies came back positive only for phenothiazines. She was seen by the on-call psychiatrist, who elicited a psychosocial history.

The patient related that she took some of her mother's tranquilizers because she wanted to die. The patient's father had abandoned the family when the patient was 3 months old. Her mother had worked as long as she could remember. At present her mother worked evenings and so they seldom saw each other. During several periods the patient was sent to live with relatives whom she did not like. Recently she began dating a boy and had grown very fond of him. Her mother disapproved of the relationship and repeatedly chastised her daughter because of it. The day before the ingestion of the pills her boyfriend had ended the relationship at least partially because of the opposition of the patient's mother. In response to the breakup the patient ingested the four chlorpromazine capsules.

Despite the seemingly trivial nature and amount of drug taken, the psychiatrist was impressed by the patient's depression, lack of support systems, lack of empathy from the still disbelieving mother, and discovery on further questioning of one prior "call for help" episode in the patient's history. At the age of 12 she had run away from home and was missing for 3 days.

The decision was made to admit the patient to the psychiatry service of the hospital for further evaluation and stabilization.

SUGGESTED READINGS

Curran BE: Suicide. *Pediatr Clin North Am* 1979;26:737.

Feldman V: Letter: Serious reactions to phenothiazines. *J Pediatr* 1976;89:163.

Rohn RD, Sarles RM, Kenny TJ, et al: Adolescents who attempt suicide. *J Pediatr* 1977;90:636.

Case 49

Fourteen-year-old Female with Vomiting and Depression

CASE PRESENTATION

A 14-year-old female is brought to the emergency department by the mother because she believes the teenager has become fat in a short period of time. She is also concerned because the patient's "stomach seems upset" as evidenced by vomiting. The mother goes on to relate that her daughter has been uncooperative and verbally abusive. In addition, her school performance deteriorates daily.

After the mother leaves the room, the patient states she has gained 10 pounds over the past 3 to 4 months. Her last period was 6 months ago. Initially the young woman denied sexual activity and vaginal discharge. Review of systems was negative. She has persistent morning sickness and has swollen enlarged breasts. Menarche was at age 10, she is gravida 0/para 0 and uses no contraception. She denies prior vaginal infection, states all immunizations are up to date, and denies any drug allergies.

Vital Signs

HR: 70 beats/min
RR: 16/min
BP: 110/80 mm Hg
T: 37.7°C (99.9°F)

Physical Examination

HEENT: Negative; fundi benign
NECK: Nontender; no masses; full range of motion; no hepato-jugular reflux; no neck vein distention; normal thyroid

CHEST: Clear; enlarged, swollen breasts
CVS: Regular rhythm; no murmur; no gallop rhythm; no rub
ABD: Normal bowel sounds; no organomegaly or masses except a large
        uterine fundus consistent with a 6-month gestation; fetal heart tones
        heard at left lower quadrant regular at 140 beats/min
GU: *Pelvis:* nonvirginal introitus; Bartholin's glands, urethra, and
        Skein's glands normal. *Cervix:* bluish and soft; internal os closed.
        Adnexae: nontender without mass. *Uterus:* large, gravid, approxi-
        mate 5 month size, and anteflexed
EXT: No cyanosis, clubbing, or edema
NEURO: Normal sensory, motor, cranial nerve, and cerebellum examination;
        oriented, depressive affect
SKIN: Clear

SUGGESTED INTERVENTIONS

1. Catheterize patient for routine urinalysis, urine culture, and urine pregnancy
   test.
2. Order blood specimens for CBC and VDRL, throat and rectal cultures for
   gonorrhea and a rubella titer.
3. Request social services consultation.
4. Consult with local child protective services.

CASE DISCUSSION

The patient was informed as to the pregnancy. In response to a question about
the father's identity the girl began to cry. When asked if she had a boyfriend, she
replied that she did not. When asked if the child's father lived with her at home she
mutely shook her head yes. The physician remarked that sometimes people we
trust take advantage of us. When further prodded she indicated that her 20-year-
old step-brother was the baby's father. Further questions revealed that he was in
fact a half-brother, not a step-brother.

The teenager may present with a complaint only marginally related to her real
concern—the pregnancy. More recently the high incidence of incest has become
widely appreciated. No longer should the physician make a diagnosis of pregnancy or venereal disease in an adolescent female without further discussing the
origin of the problem with the patient. Reporting laws in most states mandate that
sexual activity below a specified age (in California, 18 and under) is by definition
abuse and requires reporting. This of course is a double-edged sword: the reporting
theoretically will decrease ongoing abuse or incest, but it will also serve to inhibit

the patient from presenting for care or counseling regarding a pregnancy and/or sexually transmitted disease.

We will first discuss some methods of conducting an interview regarding sexual behavior and then cover the medical aspects of the problem. Many adults and teenagers are awkward when discussing sexuality. Direct questions often sound accusatory and impede the collection of information. Use of the third person technique provides support for the patient and allows the patient options in answering the question.

Once an abusive or incestuous relationship is uncovered the physician should determine what behaviors have taken place. In addition, the length of time over which the abuse has happened and the frequency are important.

Most teenagers feel guilty and will hold themselves responsible for the abusive relationship. The physician should early on mention this guilt and begin to reassure the patient.

After finishing the interview with the patient, a physical examination is done. In addition to the usual examination a pelvic examination is completed. Catheterization of the bladder immediately prior to examination of the pelvis affords an empty bladder and is the best source for urinalysis culture. Cultures for gonorrhea are taken from the rectum and cervix. *Chlamydia* culture and slide test are obtained, as is a Gram stain, all from the endocervix. If a discharge is present, a wet mount and potassium hydroxide stain will diagnosis *Trichomonas* and yeast, respectively. If the sexual abuse involves recent penetration (within 4 to 5 days), evidence should be collected as in any rape. Most states require permission (separate) for evidence collection in females aged 12 and over. Police departments will usually supply a kit for collection of evidence. If fellatio is suspected, an additional gonococcal culture of the throat should be sent.

We draw a VDRL and send a urine specimen for a pregnancy test.

If the patient has been raped, if the Gram stain of the cervix is positive for gram-negative intracytoplasmic diplococci, or if there is another reason to suspect gonorrhea, we treat with ampicillin, 3.5 g, orally, plus probenecid, 1 g. Likewise, if the urine pregnancy test is negative we offer the patient pregnancy prophylaxis. We use two Ovral® (norgestrel and ethinyl estradiol) tablets given in the emergency department and two tablets 12 hours later. This drug must be given within 72 hours of coitus. Note that LoOvral® is not effective as a postcoital contraceptive.

Finally, after appropriate social service consultation, local child protective services should be contacted. They should be used for their expertise and authority in decisions regarding intervention. They will also decide if the child remains in danger of further abuse and should be removed from the home pending court action.

When a child is placed in a foster home, medical follow-up may be compromised. Carefully written instructions for the follow-up care of the patient should be given.

SUGGESTED READINGS

Mann EM: Self-reported stresses of adolescent rape victims. *J Adolesc Health Care* 1981;2:29.

Neinstein LS, Goldenring J, Carpenter S: Nonsexual transmission of sexually transmitted diseases: An infrequent occurrence. *Pediatrics* 1984;74:67.

Rosenfeld AA: The clinical management of incest and sexual abuse of children. *JAMA* 1979;242:1761.

Fourteen-year-old Female with Abdominal Pain and Vaginal Bleeding

CASE PRESENTATION

A 14-year-old black female presented with a 5-day history of colicky lower abdominal pain and nausea, a 4-day history of light vaginal spotting, and a 1-day history of left shoulder pain. She denies dysuria or vaginal discharge. Bowel movements have been normal. She was brought in by her parents because of one episode of fainting today.

Menarche was at age 11, and menses have been regular for 2 years except for the last menstrual period, which was lighter than usual and lasted only 2 days (usually lasts 4 or 5 days). She denies sexual activity. She denies prior genital infection, practices no contraception, and is gravida 0/para 0. There is no past history of similar problems. There is no sickle cell disease.

Vital Signs

T: 37.2°C (99.0°F)
HR: 110 beats/min
RR: 30/min
BP: 85/50 mm Hg
WT: 45 kg

Physical Examination

GEN: Well-developed, well-nourished black female who is pale, in moderate distress, and nervous

HEENT: *Eyes*: PERRLA; EOM intact; normal sclera and conjunctivae; well hydrated; no icterus; normal fundi. *Ears*: normal tympanic membranes
NECK: Supple without adenopathy
CHEST: Clear to auscultation
CVS: Regular rate and rhythm with a grade II/VI systolic murmur at the left upper sternal border
ABD: Mild generalized tenderness; decreased bowel sounds; no hepatosplenomegaly or masses; moderate left lower quadrant tenderness; guarding and rebound tenderness
GU: Normal Tanner stage V external female genitalia; small amount of dark clotted blood in the vagina; cervix firm with blood extruding from external os; internal os seems closed; mild cervical motion tenderness; uterus slightly enlarged; left adnexa full and very tender. *Rectum*: normal except anterior tenderness on the right
EXT: No cyanosis, clubbing, or edema
NEURO: Alert; oriented; very anxious; normal motor, sensory, cranial nerves, cerebellar, reflex examination
SKIN: No rash, jaundice, or petechiae; good turgor; pale

SUGGESTED INTERVENTIONS

1. Administer oxygen, 3 L/min, via nasal prongs.
2. Place 2 large-bore IV lines, hooked to lactated Ringer's; run wide open until systolic blood pressure normalizes to approximately 115 mm Hg, pulse slows, and perfusion improves; place MAST suit under patient, ready for use.
3. Order blood specimen for CBC; type and cross-match 8 units of whole blood; send for β-hCG serum pregnancy test.
4. Insert Foley catheter; obtain specimen for urinalysis and urine pregnancy test; provide continuous volume monitoring.
5. Obtain cervical cultures to check for gonorrhea and chlamydial infection.
6. Request evaluation by gynecologist or surgeon stat.
7. If patient is stable, order ultrasound for pelvic study.

CASE DISCUSSION

Abdominal pain in the adolescent female can be one of the most difficult diagnostic challenges. The above case is of a 14-year-old with a ruptured ectopic pregnancy. Prompt diagnosis, stabilization, and consultation are essential, since this is a true surgical emergency with high mortality if untreated. Ectopic pregnancy is the most common cause of maternal mortality in the first trimester.

When dealing with teenagers, expect a reluctance to admit to sexual activity, especially in the presence of parents. Also, remember that the average age of initiating sexual intercourse in the United States is about 15 years of age. Teenagers should be allowed privacy when being examined, and confidentiality should be maintained whenever possible.

There is sometimes hesitation to perform pelvic examinations on children and young adolescents. It is essential, however, when pelvic pathology is in the differential diagnosis. Young teenagers and their parents are often upset and frightened by this prospect. Spending just a few minutes explaining the need for a pelvic examination and showing her the speculum will help relieve some of the patient's anxiety. Using a smaller-sized plastic speculum and performing a one-fingered vaginal examination or a rectal examination can lessen the discomfort.

The etiology of ectopic pregnancy involves conditions that delay or prevent the normal passage of the fertilized egg along the fallopian tube to the uterus. The most likely cause is infection of the pelvic organs (pelvic inflammatory disease) with *Chlamydia, Neisseria gonorrhoeae* or anaerobic and gram-negative organisms or tuberculosis. This can cause scarring and obstruction of the tubes. Previous pelvic surgery, especially of the fallopian tubes (e.g., tuboplasty, failed tubal ligation, or prior ectopic pregnancy removal), can also cause obstruction. The use of an intrauterine device may predispose to ectopic implantation, but this is debatable. Congenital anomalies of the genital tract can also increase the risk of ectopic pregnancy. Other possible causes are endometriosis, use of the progestin-only "mini pill," multiple previous therapeutic abortions, tubal mucosal motility disorders, delayed ovulation, and psychoneurogenic disorders.

Ectopic pregnancy classically presents as a missed or abnormal menstrual period, with the onset of vaginal bleeding 2 to 4 weeks later, followed, after several days, by the sudden onset of pelvic pain. This progresses to generalized abdominal pain, cervical motion tenderness, palpable adnexal mass, and, with rupture, clinical shock. However, the majority of patients have a less typical course, and the diagnosis is often initially missed. Abdominal pain is the most consistent symptom (95% to 100% of patients) and occurs unilaterally in the lower abdomen in 33% of cases, the entire abdomen in 44%, and elsewhere (shoulder, back, vagina) in 23%. Abnormal vaginal bleeding is seen in 75% of patients, amenorrhea in 70%, dizziness in 31%, nausea and vomiting in 30%, syncope in 28%, signs of pregnancy in 14%, and symptoms of urinary tract infection in 12%.

The physical examination will reveal adnexal tenderness in 95% of patients (unilateral in 60%, bilateral in 40%), abdominal tenderness in 90%, cervical motion tenderness in 50%, adnexal mass in 40% (20% of these are contralateral to the actual ectopic pregnancy!), rebound tenderness in 35%, enlarged uterus in 30%, abdominal distention in 20%, clinical shock in 17%, and fever in 7%.

The use of laboratory tests can be confusing and should not delay initiation of treatment. The hematocrit is less than 30% in only 27% of cases. The WBC count is greater than 10,000/cu mm in less than 50%. The ESR is elevated in about 15%. The pregnancy test is helpful, but remember that the serum level of hCG is lower in ectopic pregnancy than in normal pregnancy, averaging about 600 to 700 mIU/mL. Thus, the older slide pregnancy tests (e.g., Dri-Dot®) are often negative, whereas the serum pregnancy tests and the newer slide and tube urine tests are much less likely to give a false-negative result. Culdocentesis will reveal non-clotting blood with a hematocrit of greater than 15% in 90% of patients with a ruptured ectopic pregnancy. Specificity and sensitivity of culdocentesis range from 85% to 95% in various studies. Pelvic ultrasound can also be very useful in making the diagnosis, especially if an intrauterine gestational sac is seen. This makes the likelihood of a concomitant (twin) ectopic pregnancy 1:30,000! Failing this finding, the ultrasound may define a "ring sign" of concentric adnexal echos locating a possible ectopic pregnancy. Finally, free intrapelvic fluid may be detected.

The differential diagnosis of an adolescent female with acute pelvic pain should include pelvic inflammatory disease, abortion (threatened or incomplete), appendicitis, dysfunctional uterine bleeding, persistent corpus luteum cysts and other ovarian cysts, endometriosis, pyelonephritis, ovarian torsion, and mittelschmerz.

The location of an ectopic pregnancy is usually in the body of the fallopian tube (90% to 95%). Other locations are interstitial or cornual (3%), infundibular or fimbrial (3%), abdominal (1% to 2%), ovarian (1%), and cervical (less than 1%).

The emergency department treatment of ruptured ectopic pregnancy is as follows:

1. Oxygenation and establishment of good venous access.
2. Stabilization of vital signs, often requiring large amounts of fluid and blood products.
3. Confirmation of diagnosis by ultrasound if hemodynamically stable, or culdocentesis if not. Patients generally undergo laparoscopy or are operated on directly regardless of the culdocentesis finding if clinical suspicion is high and patient is hypotensive.
4. Preparation for surgery. Laparotomy with salpingectomy is the most common procedure done.

The incidence of ectopic pregnancy has increased dramatically in the past 2 decades (probably due to increasing rates of sexually transmitted diseases). It now occurs in about 1% of all pregnancies. The incidence in teenagers is about one half of this (1 in 200). Following ectopic pregnancy, infertility or repeat ectopic pregnancy occur in more than 70% of these women.

SUGGESTED READINGS

Brenner P, Roy S, Mishell D: Ectopic pregnancy: A study of 300 consecutive surgically treated cases. *JAMA* 1980;243:673.

Daling JR, Chow WH, Weiss NS, et al: Ectopic pregnancy in relation to previous induced abortion. *JAMA* 1985;253:1005–1008.

Green T: Disorders of early pregnancy. In *Gynecology—Essentials of Clinical Practice*. Boston, Little, Brown, & Co, 1977, pp 285–296.

Kitchin JD, Wein RM, Nunley WC, et al: Ectopic pregnancy: Current clinical trends. *Am J Obstet Gynecol* 1979;134:870.

Neinstein LS: Ectopic pregnancy. In Neinstein LS (ed), *Adolescent Health Care—A Practical Guide*. Baltimore, Urban and Schwarzenberg, 1984, pp 487–490.

Patrick JD: Ectopic pregnancy—a brief review. *Ann Emerg Med* 1982;11:576.

Rubin GL, Peterson HB, Dornan SF, et al: Ectopic pregnancy in the United States 1970–1978. *JAMA* 1983;249:1725.

Index